EXPECTANT MOTHERHOOD

EXPECTANT MOTHERHOOD

By

NICHOLSON J. EASTMAN, M.D.

*Professor Emeritus of Obstetrics in Johns Hopkins
University; and Obstetrician-in-Chief Emeritus
to the Johns Hopkins Hospital*

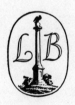

Fourth Edition, Revised

LITTLE, BROWN AND COMPANY · BOSTON · TORONTO

FOURTH EDITION

Sixth Printing

*Published simultaneously in Canada
by Little, Brown & Company (Canada) Limited*

PRINTED IN THE UNITED STATES OF AMERICA

PREFACE TO FOURTH EDITION

PREGNANCY should be a healthy, happy time. Child-bearing is a natural process, the supreme physical function of womanhood; and no other event confers so much in deep-seated, abiding contentment. As a rule, the greater span of pregnancy is associated with an increased sense of vitality and well-being. Not a few of the discomforts, which only a few decades ago were regarded as invariable accompaniments of pregnancy and labor, have been tracked to their source and are now amenable to simple preventive measures; even that old bugbear of childbirth, the pain of labor, has been so assuaged that the majority of American mothers today experience little discomfort. Meanwhile, modern methods of care have so surrounded the whole process with multiple safeguards that the likelihood of a serious complication developing is exceedingly remote.

Yes, pregnancy should be a healthy, happy time. But health and happiness in pregnancy are dependent in large measure upon proper guidance by a competent physician. There is no substitute for such advice, because it is based on personal acquaintance with the individual case. Your doctor, accordingly, should be your chief guidebook.

What, then, is the reason for a volume such as this? In the first place, it is common knowledge that intelli-

gent women of today often want more information
about the "whys" and "wherefores" of prenatal care and
labor than it is possible for the physician, in his narrow
time limits, to give them. In the second place, verbal instructions are likely to be forgotten; and since the recommendations set forth in this little book represent ac-
cepted principles of prenatal care, it is hoped that it
may serve as a sort of stenographic recapitulation of the
doctor's main instructions, which may be reviewed leisurely at home. Finally, from the viewpoint of both patient and doctor, it is hoped that many of the questions
which almost every expectant mother asks will find answer here, so that her visits to the physician may be devoted more largely to the particular circumstances of the
individual case.

*   *   *   *

Obstetrics marches on; and during the six years which
have elapsed since the third edition of *Expectant Motherhood* appeared, various improvements in maternity
care have made childbearing an even safer, more comfortable and happier experience than it was just a short
time ago. Having a baby today, provided that you are in
the hands of a competent doctor, is a much safer undertaking than a long automobile trip. And as for comfort in labor, numerous efficacious techniques of pain relief await you. Moreover, doctors and nurses everywhere
are developing a broader appreciation of the many
problems which expectant mothers face, with the result
that individual questions are answered with increasing
understanding and insight.

The meticulous attention which is being given to expectant mothers, including those in labor, is making increasing inroads on the schedules of doctors and nurses alike. Consequently they often find their time somewhat curtailed for instructing their patients in the many *routine* details of prenatal hygiene which these women should know. The reception accorded the first three editions of *Expectant Motherhood,* as well as innumerable letters from doctors and patients, has encouraged me to believe that this little book has served a useful purpose by providing this information in simple, practical form. It is likewise gratifying to be told that it has saved a certain amount of time for physicians the country over by sparing them countless questions in the office and many telephone calls both day and night.

This fourth edition of *Expectant Motherhood* incorporates the principal advances made in maternity care over recent years to the end that this small volume may continue to serve as a thoroughly modern guidebook for expectant mothers.

NICHOLSON J. EASTMAN, M.D.

Baltimore, Maryland

CONTENTS

Involution of Uterus. Meaning of Involution. — The Lochia.

Lactation. Time Relationships. — Onset of Lactation. — Quantity of Milk. — Quality of Milk. — Time of Nursing. — Care of the Nipples. — Teaching the Baby to Nurse. — Breast versus Artificial Feeding. — Rooming-in.

Hygiene of the Puerperium. Diet. — Bowels. — Bladder. — Abdominal Binder. — Visitors. — The "Baby Blues." — Afterpains. — Cracked Nipples. — Getting Up and Going Home. — Exercises. — Knee-Chest Position. — Resumption of Tub Baths. — Intercourse. — Final Examination. — Return of Menstruation. — Activities.

ILLUSTRATIONS

EXPECTANT MOTHERHOOD

Chapter I

SIGNS AND SYMPTOMS OF PREGNANCY

IN ancient Rome it was customary for a young woman after marriage to wear about her neck a snug-fitting band of some rigid material such as gold, silver or brass. These bandeaux were often exquisitely wrought, but their main purpose was not ornamental but diagnostic. From many an old wives' tale the young woman had learned that when pregnancy supervened the bandeau would become uncomfortably tight. Its removal, accordingly, carried an obvious implication and was the occasion of great rejoicing in the household, for it meant that the young woman had set forth on the Great Adventure — the creation of a new life.

Although many centuries have passed since the time of the Roman bandeau, human curiosity remains much the same and the first visit of the modern expectant mother to her doctor is usually prompted by the old query: Am I really pregnant? Oddly enough, this is the one question which the physician may answer equivocally, because even the most careful examination will rarely reveal clear-cut evidence of pregnancy until two menstrual periods have been missed, and occasionally the diagnosis may remain uncertain for a longer time. The physician bases his decision on three main types of

evidence: the patient's observation, the physical examination and, in some instances, on laboratory tests.

THE PATIENT'S OBSERVATIONS

Cessation of Menstruation. — In a healthy married
woman who has previously menstruated regularly, cessation of menstruation suggests strongly that impreg-
nation has occurred. Not until the date of the expected
period has been passed by ten days or more, however,
can any reliance be put on this symptom. Contrary to
general opinion there is scarcely a woman who menstruates exactly every twenty-eight or thirty days. This
question has been the subject of several recent studies
on normal young women, chiefly student nurses, who
have conscientiously recorded the precise time and character of each period. From these investigations it is clear
that the majority of women (almost 60 per cent) experience variations in the length of their individual cycles
which exceed five days; differences in the same woman
of even ten days are not uncommon and occur without
explanation and without apparent detriment to health.
When, however, the expected period has been passed
by more than ten days, under the circumstances mentioned, the likelihood of pregnancy is good. When the
second period is also missed, the probability naturally becomes stronger.

Although cessation of menstruation is the earliest
and one of the most important symptoms of pregnancy,
it should be noted that pregnancy may occur without
prior menstruation and that menstruation may occasion-

ally continue after conception. Several examples of the former circumstance will come to mind at once. For instance, in certain Oriental countries, where girls marry at a very early age, pregnancy frequently occurs before the menstrual periods set in; again, nursing mothers, who usually do not menstruate during the period of lactation, often conceive at this time; more rarely, women who think they have passed the menopause are startled to find themselves pregnant. Conversely, it is not uncommon for a woman to have one or two periods after conception, but almost without exception these are brief in duration and scant in amount. In such cases the first period ordinarily lasts two days instead of the usual five and the next only a few hours. Although there are instances in which women are said to have menstruated every month throughout pregnancy, these are of questionable authenticity and are probably ascribable to some abnormality of the reproductive organs. Indeed, *vaginal bleeding at any time during pregnancy should be regarded as abnormal and reported to the physician at once.*

Absence of menstruation may result from a number of conditions other than pregnancy. Probably one of the most common causes of delay in the onset of the period is psychic influence, particularly fear of pregnancy. Change of climate, exposure to cold, as well as certain chronic diseases such as anemia, may likewise suppress the menstrual flow.

Breast Changes. — Slight temporary enlargement of the breasts, causing sensations of weight and fullness, are noted by most women prior to their menstrual periods.

The earliest breast symptoms of pregnancy are merely exaggerations of these changes. Thus, the breasts become larger, firmer and more tender; a sensation of stretching fullness accompanied by tingling both in the breasts and in the nipples often develops, and in many instances a feeling of throbbing is also experienced. As time goes on, the nipple and the elevated, pigmented area immediately around it — the areola — become darker in color. The areola tends to become puffy and its diameter, which in virgins rarely exceeds an inch and a half, gradually widens to reach two or even three inches. Embedded in this areola lie tiny milk glands which take on new growth with the advent of pregnancy and appear as little protuberances, or follicles. These have been called "Montgomery's tubercles" after a famous Irish obstetrician of the nineteenth century who described them very completely and, in summarizing, created a famous medical pun by saying, "They are, in fact, a constellation of miniature nipples scattered over a milky way." These "tubercles of Montgomery" make their appearance about the eighth week of pregnancy, may not be noticed by the patient, but constitute one of the changes which the doctor will probably look for. It is needless to say that all these alterations are directed ultimately at furnishing milk for the baby, and as early as the fourth month — the time varies somewhat — a little silvery-white, sticky fluid may be expressed from the nipple; this is a watery precursor of milk, called "colostrum." During the latter part of pregnancy this fluid may be sufficient in quantity to necessitate the wearing of a small pad over the nipples to protect the clothes. At the same time it may dry on the surface of the nipples in small flakes which are often irritating and tend to make the nipples sore; if this occurs, the nipples should be gently washed with warm water, as is necessary, and then thoroughly dried. About the fifth month of pregnancy it is frequently observed that patches of brownish discoloration appear on the normal skin immediately surrounding the areola. This is known as the "secondary areola" and is an almost certain sign of pregnancy, provided the woman has never previously nursed an infant. With the increasing growth and activity of the breasts it is not surprising that a richer blood supply is needed and to this end the blood vessels supplying the area enlarge. As a result the veins beneath the skin of the breast, which previously may have been scarcely visible, now become more prominent and occasionally exhibit intertwining patterns over the whole chest wall.

In primigravidas (women pregnant for the first time) these breast changes are helpful adjuncts in the diagnosis of pregnancy, but in women who have already borne children, particularly if they have nursed an infant within the past year, they naturally are of much less significance.

Frequency of Urination. — Irritability of the bladder with resultant frequency of urination may be one of the earliest symptoms of pregnancy. It is attributed to the fact that the growing uterus stretches the base of the bladder so that a sensation results identical with that felt when the bladder wall is stretched with urine. As pregnancy progresses, the uterus rises out of the pelvis and the frequent desire to urinate subsides. Later on, however, the symptom is likely to return, for during the last weeks the head of the baby may press against the bladder and give rise to a similar condition. Although frequency of urination may be somewhat bothersome, both at the beginning and at the end of pregnancy, it should never constitute a reason for reducing the quantity of fluid consumed, which should not fall below six or eight glasses a day. If, late in pregnancy, frequency of urination disturbs sleep, the full amount of fluid should be taken before six in the evening and liquid avoided until morning.

Nausea. — About one third of pregnant women suffer no nausea whatsoever. Another third, during the early part of pregnancy, experience waves of nausea for a few hours in the morning, but this does not proceed to the point of vomiting. In the remaining third the nausea may cause actual vomiting. When this "morning sickness" occurs it usually makes its appearance about two weeks after the first missed menstrual period and subsides ordinarily after a month or six weeks. Since this symptom is present in many other conditions, such as ordinary indigestion, it is of no diagnostic value unless associated with other evidence of pregnancy.

Quickening. — This is an old term derived from an idea prevalent many years ago that at some particular moment of pregnancy life is suddenly infused into the infant. At the time this notion was in vogue, the first tangible evidence of intra-uterine life lay in the mother's feeling the baby move and the conclusion was only natural that the infant "became alive" at the moment these movements were first felt. As is reflected in the Biblical reference to the "quick and the dead," the word "quick" used to mean "alive" and the word "quickening," "becoming alive." Hence, our forebears were wont to say that when fetal movements were first felt, "quickening" or "coming to life" of the baby had occurred. We now know that the infant is a living organism from the moment of conception, but the old term "quickening" is still used in the best obstetrical circles, while among the laity "feeling life" is the common synonym. As used today, quickening refers only, of course, to the active movements of the child as first perceived by the mother.

Quickening is usually felt toward the end of the fifth month as a tremulous fluttering low in the abdomen. The first impulses caused by the stirring of the baby may be so faint as to raise some doubt as to their cause; later on, however, they grow stronger and become often so vigorous that many mothers are inclined to wonder if the baby is not destined to become an acrobat. Although quite painless, they may occasionally disturb the mother's sleep during the later weeks.

Many babies who are alive and healthy seem to move about very little in the uterus and not infrequently a day or so may pass without a movement being felt. Inability to feel the baby move does not mean that it is dead or in any way a weakling, but in all probability that it has assumed a position in which its movements are not so readily felt by the mother. Moreover, it is a well-established fact that the baby in the uterus sleeps and it seems likely that the periods of active movements and quiescence which the mother notices correspond with the phases of somnolence and wakefulness. Should three or four days pass without movements, the physician should be asked to listen for the baby's heart sounds; if these are heard it means beyond peradventure that the baby is alive and presumably in good condition. It might seem that the sensations produced by the baby's movements would be so characteristic as to make this a positive sign of pregnancy but, oddly enough, women occasionally misinterpret movements of gas in the intestines as motions of a baby and on this basis fancy themselves pregnant. The patient's statement that she feels the baby move, therefore, cannot be regarded as absolute proof of pregnancy.

Other Changes. — As pregnancy advances, possibly long after the diagnosis of the condition has been definitely established, other changes will be noted by the expectant mother. Most obvious of these, naturally, is the increasing size of the abdomen. As early as the end of the third month she may be able to feel a soft lump just above the pubic bone. This is the pregnant uterus which gradually enlarges to reach the navel at the end of the fifth month and, as shown in Figure 1, eventually fills the greater part of the abdomen. Despite the best efforts of the dressmaker at camouflage, pregnancy begins to "show" about the time the growing uterus reaches the navel, that is, at the end of the fifth month, and thereafter it is usually impossible to conceal the condition. Attempts to do so by tight lacing are dangerous, not a few serious accidents having resulted from this practice.

During the latter half of pregnancy pinkish streaks, resembling little scars, may appear over the lower abdomen. These represent small breaks in the lower layer of

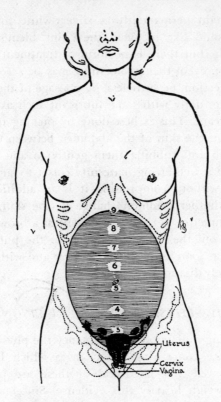

Figure 1. The Height Reached by
the Uterus at Successive Months of
Pregnancy.

the skin, which is less elastic than the upper and gives
way in places to the stretching caused by the enlarging
uterus. They are occasionally seen also on the dependent
parts of the breasts and on the thighs. After the birth
of the baby these streaks, or "striae" as physicians call

them, remain permanently as silvery-white lines. Most women would like to avoid these tiny blemishes if at all possible, but there is no form of treatment which is certain to prevent them. Something may be accomplished in this direction, nevertheless, by massage of the skin for ten minutes daily with some lubricant such as olive oil or cold cream. This is best done by picking up successive folds of the skin of the abdomen between the finger and thumb and rubbing them gently to and fro. The wearing of a well-fitting maternity corset to support the abdomen without compressing it is an additional preventive. Another common change in the skin, particularly in brunettes, is the development of a brownish line running from the navel downward to the pubic bone; this fades as soon as pregnancy is over and with time almost entirely disappears.

THE PHYSICIAN'S OBSERVATIONS

In making a diagnosis of pregnancy the physician will first inquire concerning the changes which have just been reviewed and if several of these are present is likely to weigh heavily this evidence. Since no one of these symptoms is an infallible sign of pregnancy, however, he usually lays greater stress on the results of his physical examination.

Breast Changes. — As a rule, the physician begins his examination for the determination of pregnancy by inspection of the breasts, checking up on any alterations noted by the patient, such as pigmentation, Montgomery's tubercles, etc., changes which we have described in foregoing paragraphs; in addition he may compress the nipple in an effort to demonstrate the presence of colostrum.

Fetal Heart Sounds. — The abdominal examination comprises palpation of the uterus and, if this has risen well above the pubic bone, listening for the baby's heartbeats. Of all the signs of pregnancy, hearing the sounds made by the fetal heart is the most positive, and if they are definitely heard by an experienced physician, there can be no question about the diagnosis. Curiously enough, these heart sounds were first encountered more or less by accident. Something over a hundred years ago it so happened that a Swiss physician thought it might be interesting to place his ear over the abdomen of a pregnant woman and try to hear the baby splashing about in the fluid surrounding it. Anticipating splashes, he was amazed to hear faint, rhythmic beats which resembled the ticking of a watch under a pillow, and shortly he realized that he was listening — for the first time in history — to the heartbeats of a baby within the uterus. The rate of the fetal heart is much faster than the usual rate of the maternal heart and ordinarily approximates 140 beats a minute. Under favorable circumstances these sounds become audible about the middle of the fifth month but often are not heard until several weeks later. By this time, accumulated evidence of other types has usually made the diagnosis so clear that this final proof is scarcely necessary. Nevertheless, these tick-tock messages from within the uterus, proclaiming in unequivocal terms the welfare of the baby, are always reassuring to mother and physician alike.

Fetal Movements. — Although, as we have seen, mothers may be incorrect about the sensations which they interpret as movements of the baby, the impulse which such a movement conveys to the examining hand of the physician is unmistakable and constitutes a positive sign of pregnancy. These movements, however, are usually not palpable until the end of the fifth month.

Pelvic Examination. — Since it is customary (and highly desirable) for patients to visit their physician as soon as they suspect pregnancy, the doctor is often called upon to make the diagnosis at a stage so early that fetal movements and heart sounds are not yet detectable. He accordingly supplements the evidence given by the patient and that afforded by his inspection of the breasts by an examination of the reproductive organs themselves. With the patient completely draped in a sheet and relaxed, the folds of the sheet in the region of the external reproductive organs are separated and the mucous membrane of the vagina inspected. Ordinarily this is pink in color, but early in pregnancy it acquires a dusky, bluish tinge. With two fingers of his gloved hand, the physician then carries out an internal examination in order to determine whether characteristic changes are present in the uterus itself. If the patient will close her eyes, let all her muscles "go loose," and breathe quietly through her mouth, she will not only be helping the physician, but will find that the whole procedure is quite painless. The degree to which the uterus is enlarged, its shape and consistency are all valuable diagnostic aids and when considered with the other evidence usually permit of a highly probable diagnosis of pregnancy soon after the second period has been missed.

LABORATORY TESTS

Since the very dawn of civilization efforts have been made to devise a satisfactory test for pregnancy. The priest-physicians of ancient Egypt, in the earliest writings handed down to us, tell of a test then in vogue based on the seeming ability of pregnancy urine to stimulate the growth of wheat and barley seeds; the itinerant physicians of classical Greece employed similar tests, while during the Middle Ages the omniscient physician merely gazed at the urine and in this way claimed to be able to diagnosticate not only pregnancy but many other conditions. Today, thanks to the studies of two German doctors, Aschheim and Zondek, we have at last a sound and trustworthy test for pregnancy and interestingly enough it is performed, like the tests of old, on urine. In carrying out the test a small quantity of morning urine is injected into a mouse or rabbit. If the urine comes from a pregnant woman, definite and characteristic changes are produced in the ovaries of the animal within forty-eight or seventy-two hours; if the person is not pregnant no alterations whatsoever occur. This test is accurate in about 95 per cent of cases and in the presence of pregnancy will yield a positive reaction (characteristic changes in the ovaries of the test animal) two weeks after the first missed menstrual period, sometimes earlier. It is expensive, however, quite unnecessary in most cases, and is generally performed only when the physician finds some medical reason for haste in making the diagnosis.

During recent years a similar test which makes use of the South African toad as the test animal has gained wide popularity. Within eight to eighteen hours after the urine of a pregnant woman has been injected into female toads of this variety, myriads of eggs are extruded which can be plainly seen on the floor of the aquarium in which the toads are kept. This test is often loosely referred to as the "frog test."

X-Ray Diagnosis. — The skeleton of the growing baby is usually demonstrable in X-ray pictures of the mother's abdomen from the beginning of the fifth month and when thus seen is, of course, absolute proof of pregnancy. Visualization of the infant is rarely possible before the middle of the fourth month (fourteen weeks); since by this time other types of evidence are usually conclusive, the X-ray is little used in the diagnosis of pregnancy.

In summary, then, the earliest symptoms of pregnancy are cessation of menstruation, enlargement of the breasts, frequency of urination and nausea. Although none of these is absolute proof of pregnancy, cessation of menstruation followed by one or more of the other symptoms is strongly suggestive; if two periods are missed and any of the other symptoms are also present, pregnancy is highly probable. Unless the mouse, rabbit, or frog test is used, the physician is unable, as a rule, to make a clear-cut diagnosis until after the second missed period and in some cases it is impossible until after the third missed period. Absolute proof of pregnancy, if you are skeptical of these "probable diagnoses," must await the fifth month when the baby's heart sounds become audible, when its movements begin to be palpable by the physician, and when its bony structure is demonstrable by the X-ray.

Chapter II

GROWTH AND DEVELOPMENT
OF THE FETUS

IN all Nature's wide universe of miracles there is no process more wondrous, no mechanism more incredibly fantastic, than the one by which a tiny speck of tissue, the human egg, develops into a crying, seven-pound baby. So miraculous did primitive peoples consider this phenomenon that they ascribed it all to superhuman intervention and even overlooked the fact that sexual intercourse was a necessary precursor. At this very moment certain primitive tribes in East Australia believe that female babies are created by Bahloo, the moon, while male infants are fashioned at a near-by boy factory supervised by Boomayahmayahmul, the wood lizard. According to their belief, the babies, after being created in spirit by these woodland deities, suspend themselves on certain coolalabah trees whence they enter — more or less promiscuously — the bodies of passing women and there become incarnated. It is not surprising to note further that the women of this tribe, when they see a whirlwind coming, cover themselves with blankets and avoid drooping coolalabah trees!

Throughout unremembered ages our own primitive ancestors doubtless held similar beliefs, but now we know that pregnancy comes about in only one way:

from the union of a female germ cell, the egg or ovum, with a male germ cell, the spermatozoon. The former are produced, at the rate of one a month, by one or the other of the ovaries, whitish, almond-shaped bodies which lie near the uterus (see Figure 2). The process by which an ovum and a spermatozoon fuse is called by scientists "fertilization" and by the laity "conception." After an egg has been fertilized it naturally requires, like any other egg, a nest or bed in which to grow. Since a rich bed is essential to the welfare of the fertilized ovum, let us consider how it is formed each month and, in passing, take time to explain that herein lies the reason why women menstruate.

Role of Menstruation in Childbearing. — It is well known that the span of years during which childbearing is usually possible, let us say from the age of thirteen to that of forty-five, corresponds to the period during which menstruation occurs; in general, moreover, a woman who menstruates is able to conceive whereas one who does not is sterile. There is good reason for believing, therefore, that these two phenomena are closely interlinked and, since no process of Nature is purposeless, that menstruation must play some vital and indispensable role in childbearing.

The organ of menstruation, of course, is the womb or, as physicians call it, the uterus — a hollow, pear-shaped, muscular organ which in the nonpregnant state measures about three inches and is joined to the upper end of the vagina in the pelvic cavity. If, day by day, we were privileged to watch the lining membrane of this organ, we should observe some remarkable alterations. Immediately following the termination of a menstrual period, this membrane is very thin, measuring perhaps a

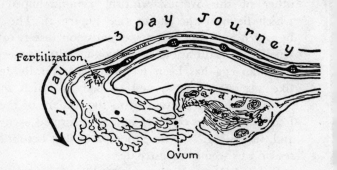

twentieth of an inch in depth. Each day thereafter it becomes a trifle thicker and harbors an increasing content of blood, while its glands become more and more active, secreting a rich nutritive substance which used to be called "uterine milk." About a week before the onset of the next expected period this process reaches its height; the lining membrane of the uterus is now the thickness of heavy, downy velvet and has become soft and succulent with blood and glandular secretions. It is at this time and into this luxuriant bed that the egg, if one has been fertilized, sinks.

All these changes have but one purpose, to provide a suitable bed in which the fertilized ovum may rest, secure nourishment and grow. Now, if an egg is not fertilized, these alterations are unnecessary and accordingly, through a mechanism which even today is obscure, the swollen lining of the uterus disintegrates, the

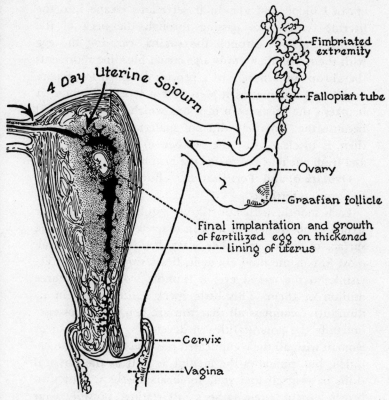

Figure 2. Showing, on the Left, the Path Followed by the Egg in Its Transit from Ovary to Uterus (the Ovary, Fallopian Tube and Uterus Having Been Laid Open for Illustrative Purposes); in the Center, a Two-Months' Pregnancy Implanted on the Thickened Uterine Lining; on the Right, the Fallopian Tube and Ovary as They Exist in the Body.

encased blood and glandular secretions escape into the uterine cavity and, passing through the neck of the uterus, flow out through the vagina, carrying the egg with them. In other words, menstrual bleeding represents the abrupt termination of a process designed to prepare board and lodging, as it were, for a fertilized ovum; it betokens the breakdown of a bed which was not needed because the "boarder" did not materialize; its purpose, then, is to clear away the old bed in order that a new and fresh one may be created the next month.

Ovulation and Fertilization. — But what happens if the ovum *is* fertilized?

Each month, with punctilious regularity, a blisterlike structure about half an inch in diameter develops on the surface of one or the other ovary. Inside this bubble, almost lost in the fluid about it, lies a tiny speck, scarcely visible to the naked eye; a thimble would hold three million of them. This little speck contains within its diminutive compass all that you are heir to; it possesses not only the potentialities of developing into a man or woman with all the complicated physical organization entailed, but embodies the mental as well as the physical traits of yourself and your forebears: perhaps your own brown eyes or your father's tall stature, possibly your mother's love of music or your grandfather's genius at mathematics. These, and a million other potentialities, are all wrapped up in this little speck, or ovum, so small that it is about one fourth the size of the period at the end of this sentence.

With the exact periodicity which characterizes so many of Nature's works, one blister on one ovary bursts at a definite time each month and discharges an ovum, a process known as ovulation. The precise day on which ovulation occurs is a matter of no small importance. For instance, since the ovum can be fertilized only within the twenty-four-hour period after its escape from the ovary, this is the only time at which a woman is really fertile. During the rest of the monthly cycle, theoretically at least, it is impossible for her to conceive. Evidence of various sorts indicates that ovulation usually occurs between the tenth and fourteenth day of the menstrual cycle, counting from the day on which bleeding begins; ordinarily, then, the most fertile time is about a week after the cessation of menstruation. While this is the rule there are many exceptions and ovulation may take place at any time between the ninth and eighteenth days of the cycle. The fact that ovulation rarely occurs during the last ten days of a twenty-eight-day cycle has given rise to the birth-control doctrine of the "Safe Period," according to which it is impossible for a child to be conceived after the eighteenth day. Theoretically, this claim is altogether sound; practically, not a few women appear to have conceived during this period so that it would seem that ovulation may occasionally take place later than theory would have us believe.

After the ovum has been discharged from the ovary it faces a perilous seven-day journey (Figure 2). Its goal is the cavity of the uterus, more than three inches away. The only pathway of approach is the tortuous Fallopian tube whose lining is wrinkled unevenly into countless little hills and valleys, and whose passageway at the inner end is no larger than a bristle. The ovum, moreover, has no means of locomotion itself but must depend on "hitchhiking" a ride, as it were, through this winding, bumpy tunnel. Offhand, it would seem an impossible feat; actually the ovum is not only able to make this journey with apparent ease but has been known to reach its destination after the most unbelievable meanderings. For instance, if one Fallopian tube has been removed by an operation the ovum may migrate to the opposite side of the uterus and enter the other tube. This whole "transportation system" is made possible, it seems, because of currents in the film of fluid which bathes the lining of the Fallopian tube. If we could inspect this lining with a microscope, we should see little hairlike projections, called cilia, which wave or beat in such a way as to direct any overlying fluid (as well as any particle afloat thereon) in the direction of the uterine cavity. Once the ovum has been expelled from the ovary it is drawn by the currents into the funnel-like opening of the tube and is thence propelled down the tube by these same currents, as well as by the muscular action of the tubal walls. But it is scarcely a third the way down the tube when the supreme event happens: it meets a spermatozoon and a new human being is created. As Miss Margaret Shea Gilbert has so happily expressed it in her book, *Biography of the Unborn,* "Life begins for each of us at an unfelt, unknown, and unhonored instant when a minute, wriggling sperm plunges headlong into a mature ovum or egg."

These minute, wriggling spermatozoa are in some respects even more remarkable than the ova which they fertilize. In appearance they resemble microscopic tadpoles, with oval heads and long lashing tails about ten times the length of the head. As is shown in Figure 3, they are much smaller than the ovum, their over-all length measuring about one quarter the diameter of the egg, and it has been estimated that the heads of two billion of them — enough to regenerate the entire population of the world — could be placed, with room to

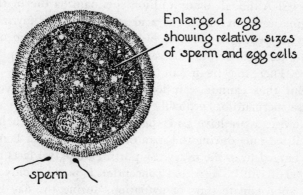

Enlarged egg showing relative sizes of sperm and egg cells

sperm

Figure 3. Relative Sizes of Egg and Spermatozoon.

spare, in the hull of a grain of rice. As a result of the wriggling motion of their tails, spermatozoa swim with a quick vibratory motion and have been "timed" under the microscope at rates as fast as one seventh of an inch a minute. In ascending the uterus and Fallopian tube they must swim against the same currents that waft the ovum downward, but nevertheless they seem able to reach the outer part of the tube within an hour or two.

Perhaps the most amazing feature of spermatozoa is their huge number. At each ejaculation, the climax of intercourse in the male, about three hundred million are discharged; if each of these could be united with an ovum, the babies which would thus be started would exceed the total number born in the United States during the past one hundred years — all from a single ejaculation. So lavish is Nature in her effort to perpetuate the species! Although many million spermatozoa die in the vagina as the result of the acid secretion there, myriads survive, penetrate the neck of the uterus and swarm upward through the uterine cavity and into the Fallopian tube. There they lie in wait for the ovum.

But they cannot wait long for they are short-lived, these spermatozoa, probably not living over a day or so. Likewise, as we have said, the ovum is capable of being fertilized only during the span of a day or so after being discharged from the ovary. By putting these two facts together it will be seen that conception is possible only at the approximate time of ovulation, during the day before or during the day or two after.

Such an important process as the union of the sperm and ovum — a mechanism upon which all future generations devolve — is not left to mere chance but is motivated by a deep-rooted quality which all germ cells of opposite sex exhibit, namely, a violent attraction toward each other. As soon as the ovum comes near the army of spermatozoa, the latter, as if they were tiny bits of steel drawn by a powerful magnet, fly at the ovum. One penetrates, but only one. By what mechanism the countless other sperms are prevented from entering the ovum is not known, but it is well-established that as soon as one enters, the door is shut on other suitors. Now, as if electrified, all the particles which make up the ovum (now fused with the sperm) exhibit vigorous agitation, as if they were being rapidly churned about by some unseen force; this becomes more and more violent until it amounts to such an upheaval that the fertilized ovum divides into two cells. This process is repeated again and again, until masses containing sixteen, thirty-two and sixty-four cells are successively produced, and so on endlessly. Meanwhile this growing aggregation of cells is being carried down the Fallopian tube in the direction of the uterine cavity.

The Determination of Sex. — If we could examine an ovum and a sperm-head through a high-powered microscope, we should find that both these cells contain a certain number of dark, oval or cylindrical bodies which stand out sharply against the surrounding tissues. These are known as chromosomes, are the carriers of hereditary characteristics and determine also, as we shall see, the sex of the embryo. Were we to examine a large number of ova just as the spermatozoa are about to enter them, we should find that each ovum contains exactly twenty-three chromosomes; but close study would reveal that one of these differs from all the rest in appearance and is known by scientists to be a carrier of sex. This atypical, sex chromosome in the ovum is called the "X" chromosome. Likewise, in the sperm we would find twenty-two chromosomes plus an atypical, sex chromosome; but here we would note that the sex chromosomes are of two types, one of which is called the "X" chromosome and the other the "Y" chromosome. Thanks to the studies of many scientists, who have examined these bodies in the utmost detail, we now know that when a sperm with an "X" chromosome fertilizes an ovum, a female infant results, while a sperm with a "Y" chromosome produces a male. The sex of the future child is then ordained the very instant the spermatozoon penetrates the ovum and depends solely on the type of sex chromosome which that particular sperm-head happens to possess. Since the number of spermatozoa containing the "Y" chromosome (boys) is of the same order as those containing the "X" (girls), the sex of the infant is a matter of sheer chance with the odds about even in the case of full-term children; actually they are slightly in favor of boys by about 106 to 100. In any event, it is the germ cell of the father, the spermatozoon, which determines the sex of the future baby; the germ cell of the mother, the ovum, can grow into either a boy or a girl — a fact well worth mentioning to any husband who is disappointed by the sex of the child! Although many attempts have been made to influence Nature's roulette wheel of sex, to the end that a child of a desired sex may be had, no success has been met. Nor can a physician predict with any degree of assurance and safety, even late in pregnancy, whether the baby will be a girl or a boy. To be sure, there are ways and means by which he may speculate, but this amounts to little more than guessing, with even chances of being right. Obviously, when the two sex cells unite, the resulting cell contains forty-six chromosomes, the number present in all the cells of the normal human body except for the sex cells which, as stated, contain twenty-three.

Embedding of the Ovum. — The journey of the ovum down the Fallopian tube is believed to require about three days; meanwhile the process of cell multiplication has proceeded to such a degree that the egg, upon entering the uterine cavity, has become a little cluster of cells not unlike a mulberry in conformation. Now, as if to rest on its oars, the ovum spends a leisurely sojourn of some four days in the uterine cavity, apparently doing nothing. Internally, nevertheless, important changes are taking place. The cells in the center of the mulberry mass secrete a fluid which pushes the remaining cells to the periphery of the sphere. At the same time it becomes apparent that this external envelope of cells is actually made up of two different layers, an inner and an outer. A specialized portion of the inner layer, after some 260 days, will develop into the long-awaited baby. The outer layer is a sort of foraging unit, called the "trophoblast," which means "feeding" layer; it is the principal function of these cells to secure food for the embryo.

While the ovum is undergoing these changes, the lining of the uterus, it will be recalled, is making preparations for its reception. Considering that ovulation took place on the fourteenth day of the menstrual cycle and that the tubal journey and the uterine sojourn required three and four days, respectively, twenty-one days of the cycle will have passed before the ovum has developed its trophoblastic layer of cells. As we have seen, this is just the period when the lining of the uterus has reached its the greatest thickness and succulence. In other words, timing has been precisely correct; the bed is prepared and the ovum has so developed that it is now ready to dig into that bed.

The embedding of the ovum is the work of the outer "foraging" layer of cells, the trophoblast, which possesses the peculiar property of being able to digest or liquefy the tissues with which it comes into contact. In this manner these cells not only burrow into the uterine lining and eat out a nest for the ovum, but also digest the walls of the many small blood vessels which they encounter beneath the surface. The mother's blood stream is thus tapped and presently the ovum finds itself deeply sunk in the lining bed of the uterus, with tiny pools of blood around it. Sprouting out from the trophoblastic layer, quivering, fingerlike projections now develop and extend greedily into the blood-filled spaces. For the next nine months these fingerlike sprouts serve the fetus as lungs and digestive organs. Through them oxygen, water and simple foodstuffs, such as sugar and calcium, pass from mother to child, while in the opposite direction the waste products of the fetus diffuse. At no time, it must be understood, does the blood of the mother mingle with that of the fetus; the maternal blood bathes the outside of the trophoblastic projections, the fetal circulation courses within them, and any substances which pass from one blood to the other must permeate the walls of these structures.

The Bag of Waters and Afterbirth. — With the nutritional facilities thus provided, the cells which are destined to form the baby grow rapidly. At first they all look alike but soon after embedding, groups of cells here and there assume distinctive characteristics; some develop into bone, some into skin, others into heart, blood vessels, etc. Even before these structures become evident, however, a fluid-filled space develops about the embryo, a space which is lined with a smooth, slippery membrane; this, in turn, is surrounded by another thicker and stronger membrane. The space is the amniotic cavity, while the membranes and the fluid they contain are often spoken of as the "bag of waters," in which the fetus floats and moves about. The amniotic fluid has a number of important functions. It keeps the fetus at an even temperature, cushions it against possible injury and provides a medium in which it can move about easily; it is known, furthermore, that the fetus drinks this fluid. At the end of the fourth month of pregnancy the bag of waters has enlarged to the size of a large orange and occupies the entire interior of the uterus.

Meanwhile another important structure has formed, the afterbirth. This is a fleshy, disclike organ which late in pregnancy measures about eight inches in diameter and one inch in thickness. It receives its name from the fact that its birth follows after that of the child; physicians refer to it as the "placenta," a term derived from the Latin word for cake, which it resembles in shape. The afterbirth, or placenta, is formed by the union of the fingerlike projections of the trophoblast and the lining bed of the uterus into which they sink. An analogous situation is seen when a tree or plant sends down its roots into a bed of earth for nourishment; when the plant is removed a certain amount of the earthy bed clings to the interlocking roots. Similarly, a thin layer

of the uterine bed clings to the branching projections of
trophoblast and together they make up this organ which
supplies food to the baby just as the roots and earth
provide nourishment for a plant. The placenta is connected to the fetus by means of the umbilical cord, a
gelatinous, coiling structure about twenty inches long.
Within it are vessels whose blood carries oxygen and
food from placenta to fetus and waste products from
fetus to placenta.

The Development of the Baby Month by Month. —
Most women consider themselves one month pregnant at
the time of the first missed menstrual period, two months
pregnant at the second missed period, and so on. Since
conception does not ordinarily take place until some fourteen days after the onset of menstruation, it is obvious
that an embryo does not attain the age of one month
until about a fortnight after the first missed period
(assuming a twenty-eight-day cycle) and its "birthday" by
months regularly falls two weeks or so after any numeric-
ally specified missed period. This should be remembered
in reading the month-by-month development of the fetus
below. In thus speaking of the age of a pregnancy in
"months," physicians refer to "lunar months," that is,
periods of four weeks. Since a lunar month corresponds
to the usual length of the menstrual cycle they find it
easier to "figure" in this way.

Month by month the development of the fetus is somewhat as follows:

End of First Lunar Month (Figure 4). The embryo is
about one quarter of an inch long if measured in a
straight line from head to tail — for we do have tails at

this early stage. The backbone has been laid down but is so bent upon itself that the head almost touches the tip of the tail. At one end of the backbone the head is extremely prominent, representing almost one third of the entire embryo. (Throughout intra-uterine life the head is always very large in proportion to the body, a relationship which is still present, although to a lesser degree, at birth.) The tube which will form the future heart has been formed and produces a large, rounded bulge on the body wall; even at this early date this structure is pulsating regularly and propelling blood through microscopic arteries. The rudiments of the future digestive tract are also discernible — a long, slender tube leading from the mouth to an expansion in the same tube which will become the stomach; connected with the latter the beginnings of the intestines may be seen. The incipient arms and legs are represented by small budlike nubbins.

End of Second Lunar Month (Figure 4). The embryo now begins to assume human form and hereafter until birth is referred to as a "fetus." He has an unmistakably human face, and also arms and legs, with fingers, toes, elbows and knees. During the past four weeks he has quadrupled in length and measures about one inch from head to buttocks; his weight is approximately one thirtieth of an ounce. The sex organs become apparent but it is difficult to distinguish between male and female. It is during the second month that the human tail reaches its greatest development, but by the end of the month it is less prominent and thereafter undergoes retrogression.

End of Third Lunar Month (Figure 4). The fetus now measures somewhat over three inches in length and weighs an ounce. The sex can now be distinguished by the presence or absence of the uterus. The finger- and toenails appear as fine membranes. Early in this month buds for all the temporary "baby" teeth are laid down and sockets for these develop in the jawbone. A rudimentary kidney has developed and secretes small amounts of urine into the bladder which in all probability escape later into the amniotic fluid. Movements of the fetus are known to occur at this time but are too weak to be felt by the mother.

End of Fourth Lunar Month (Figure 5). The fetus from head to toe is now six and a half inches long and about four ounces in weight. A fine, downy growth of hair appears on the skin (so-called lanugo hair) and perhaps a few hairs on the scalp. At the end of this period faint movements of the fetus (quickening) may be felt by the mother but usually these are not experienced until the next month.

End of Fifth Lunar Month. The length of the fetus approximates ten inches while its weight is about eight ounces. It is at this period that the physician is often able to hear the fetal heart for the first time and that the mother, as we have noted, first feels the baby move. If a fetus is born now it may make a few efforts to breathe but its lungs are insufficiently developed to cope with conditions outside the uterus and it invariably succumbs within a few hours at most.

End of Sixth Lunar Month. The length of the fetus is twelve inches, and its weight a pound and a half. It re-

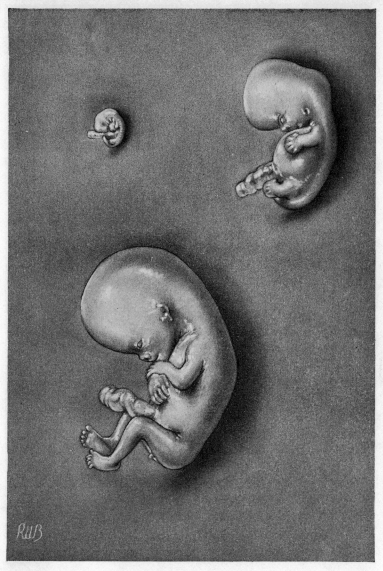

Figure 4. Actual Size of Fetus at One Month, Two Months
and Three Months.

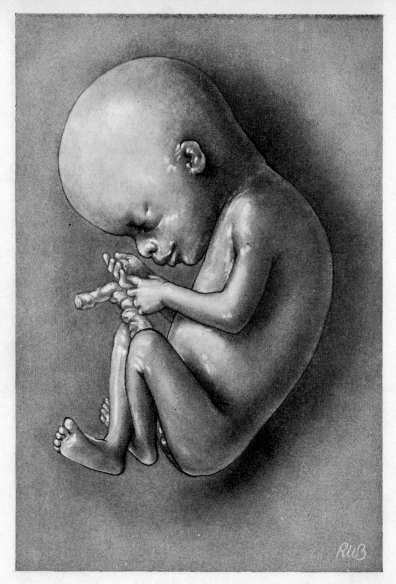

Figure 5. Actual Size of Fetus at Four Months.

sembles now a miniature baby with the exception of the skin which is wrinkled and red with practically no fat beneath it. At this time, however, the skin begins to develop a protective covering called "vernix caseosa," which means "cheesy varnish." This fatty, cheesy substance adheres to the skin of the fetus and at term may be an eighth of an inch thick. Although one or two rare cases are on record in which fetuses of this size are said to have survived, the outlook must be regarded as practically hopeless.

End of Seventh Lunar Month. The fetus measures about fifteen inches in length and weighs approximately two and a half pounds. If born at this time it has some chance of survival, perhaps one in ten. There is a widespread notion, quite incorrect, that infants born at the seventh month are more likely to survive than those born at the eighth month. This is another of those old superstitions which have descended through more than two thousand years from the time of the ancient Greek physicians. They believed that the fetus is born by means of its own effort, that is, it pushes with its legs against the upper part of the uterus and wriggles out into the world. It was their opinion that the fetus first attempts to escape from the uterus at the seventh month and if strong, it succeeds. If the attempt fails, it is repeated at the eighth month. However, if it now succeeds it is so exhausted as the result of the previous attempt that it is more likely to die than if it had been successful in the prior attempt a month earlier. We now know, of course, that the fetus is entirely passive, that it is expelled from the mother's body solely through the muscular action of the uterus and that this old belief is wholly fallacious. The fetus born at the eighth month stands a much better chance of survival than one born at the seventh.

End of Eighth Lunar Month. The fetus measures about sixteen and a half inches and weighs some four pounds. With good care infants born at the end of the eighth month have better than even chances of survival, possibly as high as two chances out of three.

End of Ninth Lunar Month. For all practical purposes the fetus is now a mature infant, measures some nineteen inches, and weighs around six pounds. As if to improve its appearance before making its debut into the world, the fetus devotes the last two months in the uterus to putting on weight and during this period gains a half pound a week. Its chances of survival are now quite as good as if born at full term.

Middle of Tenth Lunar Month. Full term has now been reached and the fetus weighs on an average about seven pounds if a girl and seven and a half if a boy; its length approximates twenty inches. Its skin is now white or pink and thickly coated with the cheesy vernix. The fine, downy hair which previously covered its body has largely disappeared. The fingernails are firm and protrude beyond the end of the fingers. The breasts in both boys and girls are often firm and protruding due to the fact that the same substance which causes the mother's breasts to enlarge during pregnancy passes through the placenta and stimulates development of the fetal breasts. This enlargement subsides within a few days after birth.

Duration of Pregnancy. — The length of pregnancy

varies greatly; it may range, indeed, between such wide extremes as 240 days and 300 days, and yet be entirely normal in every respect. The average duration, counting from the time of conception, is nine and a half lunar months, that is, thirty-eight weeks, or 266 days. Counting from the first day of the last menstrual period, its average length is ten lunar months, or forty weeks or 280 days. That these average figures mean very little, however, is shown by the following facts. Scarcely one pregnancy in ten terminates exactly 280 days after the beginning of the last period. Less than one half terminate within one week of this 280th day. In 10 per cent of cases birth occurs a week or more before the theoretical end of pregnancy and in another 10 per cent it takes place more than two weeks later than we would expect from the average figures cited above. Indeed, it would appear that some children require a longer time, others a shorter time in the uterus for full development.

Calculation of the Expected Date of Confinement. — In view of the wide variation in the length of pregnancy it is obviously impossible to predict the expected day of confinement with any degree of precision. The time-honored method, based on the above "average figures," is simple. Count back three calendar months from the first day of the last menstrual period and add seven days. For instance, if the last menstrual period began on June 10, we would count back three months to March and, adding seven days, arrive at the date of March 17. While it may be satisfying to the curiosity to have this date in mind, it must be understood that the likelihood of labor's occurring even within a week of this day is less than

50 per cent. There is one chance in ten that it will come at least two weeks later.

And yet, whether pregnancy terminates a week before or two weeks later than the day calculated, the outlook for mother and child is usually just as good as if it had ended at high noon on the due date. Actually, women seldom go "over-term"; in most of these cases it is the above system of calculation and not Nature which has erred. For example, ovulation and hence conception may have occurred some days later than usual; this would throw both the beginning and the end of pregnancy just that many days later. If, superimposed on this circumstance, we were dealing with a child which required a slightly longer stay in the uterus for complete development, it would be clear that the apparent delay was quite normal and for the best.

Maternal Impressions. — No discussion of the growth and development of the baby would be complete without consideration of the old belief that the mental condition of the mother may modify the development of the unborn infant, or, as they used to say, "mark" it. Many a young woman, with commendable determination, has set her facial muscles into a constant grin for nine long months because certain well-intentioned elders have told her that a cheerful attitude on her part ensured a cheerful disposition in her offspring. Many another has drummed the piano keys until her ears ached, in the hope that her child would be "musically gifted." Others have stayed home from the circus, in the fear that some animal might frighten them and in this way cause the baby to be "marked" or distorted in the likeness of the ugly beast.

This belief, like most obstetric superstitions, is of hoary antiquity: the Biblical story of Jacob and the "speckled and spotted kine" reflects it, while dramatists and novelists from Shakespeare to Dickens have perpetuated the idea in stirring plots. The facts are these. There is not the slightest nervous connection between mother and child; in other words, no possible pathways along which any such impulses, pleasant or otherwise, could travel. The blood of the mother is likewise separate and distinct from that of the child. Furthermore, the infant is completely formed at the end of the sixth week of pregnancy, that is, at a period when most women scarcely realize they are pregnant; and, almost without exception, the causative mental shock or experience which is alleged to have brought about the "marking" occurred much later, long after the organ in question was in its final state of formation. Lastly, all modern experience refutes the belief. Obstetricians of vast experience, as well as maternity hospitals whose annual deliveries run into the thousands, are unanimous in asserting that they have never seen an authentic case.

How, then, are we to explain this age-old superstition? A number of factors are probably at the root of it, chief among which must be listed pure coincidence. One baby in every fifty, approximately, is born with some kind of blemish. (If this worries you in the slightest, remember that ninety-eight babies out of every hundred are formed perfectly.) In the event that such a blemish is

present — let us say a reddish blotch on the buttock of
the baby — would it not be easy for an introspective
mother, who had been told of this legend, to think
finally of some object, some animal, or possibly some
article of diet she craved during pregnancy and, in her
imagination, correlate it with the little red blotch? As for
the desirability of cheerfulness during pregnancy, this
should follow naturally from the fact that you are well
and are approaching what will prove to be (although
you may not appreciate it now) the most permanently
satisfying event in your life. Do not think, however,
though you devote all your days to laughter, or all your
nights to symphony concerts, that your child will be one
bit cheerier or one whit more musical because of it. No,
his mental characteristics are more deeply rooted than
that; as we have seen, they were determined in good
measure when his grandparents married, before you and
your husband were born; and nothing you think, see or
hear during pregnancy will affect them in the slightest.

Chapter III

DIET AND HYGIENE IN PREGNANCY

THE Chinese count a person's age not from the day of birth but from the time of conception, a good way of reminding the expectant mother that all this time a living, human creature is being nourished, who will soon be "nine months old." During this vital, formative period the child is in greater need of proper nourishment and suitable environment than at any other time in his life. His well-being in this period depends, naturally, upon the health of the mother; his well-being in the years to come, moreover, as well as that of the mother, is based in substantial degree on her condition during the prenatal months. Accordingly, you can confer no greater boon on your unborn child or on your own future welfare than by placing yourself at the earliest possible moment in the hands of a competent physician. He will have many helpful suggestions about the kinds of food which should be eaten to ensure the growth of a robust baby and about the sort of routine which is most conducive to its normal development. By judicious and timely advice regarding details of personal hygiene he can do much to obviate minor discomforts and to prevent them from developing into menacing complications. His directions about maintaining the highest standards of health will impose no serious deprivations; in fact, the program recommended will resolve itself into little more than a normal, wholesome life with particular attention to food, water drinking, elimination, exercise, rest and sleep — a few of the things about which we are all so likely to forget.

The First Visit to the Physician. — Most women dread the first visit to the doctor but almost without exception they complete it with the feeling that this dread was wholly unnecessary. Physicians are not unaware that the young woman is undergoing what is probably the most intimate examination she has ever experienced and they strive in every way to protect innate modesty and prevent unnecessary exposure by the use of sheets and other drapings. There is no pain involved in any of the procedures.

The physician first inquires into your past health and that of your parents and husband. His purpose in so doing is to ascertain whether there are any past illnesses or hereditary tendencies which might be lighted up by pregnancy, and if so, he institutes precautionary measures. If there have been previous pregnancies, he reviews these searchingly. Since menstruation is so closely associated with childbearing, he has several questions to ask about the past menstrual history; and in order to fix some approximate date for the expected confinement, he notes the date of the last period.

The greater part of the examination is identical with that which any thorough physician carries out on any patient. As a rule the first item on the program is to step on the scales and be weighed. The physician will then put a cuff on your upper arm and take the blood-pressure reading. This is one part of the examination, and almost the only one, which will have to be repeated at subsequent visits. It is a procedure of the utmost importance since a rise in blood pressure is the very earliest sign of a common complication, toxemia of pregnancy, concerning which we shall hear more later. The teeth and throat are then inspected, followed possibly by a suggestion to visit the dentist in the near future. The chest is then tapped and listened to with a stethoscope to make sure that the heart and lungs are normal. Examination of the breasts is important for two reasons: first, in early cases, to secure confirmatory evidence of the existence of pregnancy, as we have seen in Chapter I; and second, to ascertain whether the nipples seem satisfactory for nursing; if they are not, certain simple manipulative procedures may be recommended. Examination of the abdomen varies with the duration of pregnancy. If you have visited the doctor early (as every woman should), he will simply make note of its general contour, whether the wall is firm or flabby, and so forth. If you are further along, the size of the uterus is recorded, the position of the baby determined, and its heart sounds listened to. The abdominal examination is usually repeated at subsequent visits, particularly during the later months, because it is naturally important for the doctor to know that the baby is doing well (heart sounds) and lies in a favorable position.

Labor, the process by which the baby is born, resolves itself largely into the passage of the infant through a bony canal, the pelvis; and it goes without saying that if labor is to proceed smoothly, this canal must be of adequate size. Exact measurement of the pelvis is therefore most important. Except for the fact that calipers, rather than a tape measure, are used, this procedure is not unlike that which any dressmaker might employ in measuring the size of the hips. After all, however, it is the inside of the pelvis through which the baby must pass and one internal examination, to make sure that the internal measurements are ample, must be done at some time in the prenatal course. Many physicians carry this out at the first visit while others defer it until a later time. In any event, as we have already said, if you relax, the internal examination is not painful and will be over in a few seconds.

Finally, as a rule, a small sample of blood is taken by puncturing a vein on the upper arm with a fine needle attached to a syringe. This "stick" is avowedly unpleasant but the discomfort is momentary, and a careful study of the blood is desirable for several reasons. In the first place, as a result of the fact that the fetus and growing uterus consume a great amount of iron, the substance out of which hemoglobin or the red coloring matter of our blood is built, many pregnant women develop anemia, that is, impoverishment of the blood. If the hemoglobin concentration in the blood is low, it is most important that the doctor should know the fact since the addition of a little iron to the diet will ordinarily remedy the condition in a short time. Another purpose in examining the blood of the prospective mother is to determine the Wassermann reaction, in other words, to rule out the presence of syphilis. Ten years ago this disease was among the "unmentionables" and even to hint that a patient might have it constituted a grave offense. Although the majority of cases of syphilis are due to illicit sexual relationships, we realize today that a certain number of cases are traceable to other means of exposure such as kissing and the use of public drinking cups — the so-called "syphilis of the innocent." A person may acquire the infection in this way and be quite unaware of its presence, since many years may pass before it gives rise to serious symptoms. Nor does it seem to affect the apparent well-being of the pregnant woman. Its effect on the unborn child, however, is disastrous. The disease passes to the fetus through the placenta shortly after the middle of pregnancy has been reached; the fetus usually succumbs and the premature delivery of a dead child follows. If it is born alive it is very likely to be so feeble that it dies in the first few days or weeks of life. Even if the child survives this period, it still harbors the infection and becomes the victim of various manifestations of the disease later on. Although this picture is very distressing, it is gratifying to know that the treatment of syphilis in the pregnant woman exerts a particularly beneficial effect on the unborn child and if the treatment has been adequate the infant frequently escapes unscathed. During recent years public-health officials have shown growing concern about the prevalence of syphilis in the United States and have emphasized the ravages it is likely to work on generations to come. As a result, several states refuse to grant marriage licenses until both parties are proved to be free of syphilis by means of the Wassermann test.

While the patient is dressing, the physician goes to his laboratory and devotes these few minutes to an analysis of the urine. It is the custom of some doctors to ask their patients to bring a morning sample of urine at each visit; others provide arrangements for the patient to furnish a fresh sample in the office lavatory. The urine, like the blood pressure, sometimes shows alterations which warn of impending toxemia and is examined at each visit.

Subsequent Visits to the Physician. — In the early months of pregnancy, one visit a month to the doctor is ordinarily adequate. During the last half more frequent examinations are desirable, let us say every two or three weeks, and during the last month possibly every week. At these visits, after asking about your general well-being, the physician measures your blood pressure, analyzes the urine and records the weight. Some doctors carry out abdominal examinations on each of these occasions, while others do so only during the last two months. As a rule physicians do not charge for these individual visits but include this service (regardless of the number of office visits) in their fee for delivery. This allows you complete freedom to telephone or visit the doctor whenever symptoms warrant it, without consideration of expense; at the same time it removes a certain hesitation which the physician might have in requesting more frequent visits than usual.

There is no substitute for the individual advice and instruction which you will receive on these visits to your physician. While the following suggestions in regard to prenatal diet and hygiene are applicable in most cases, there are circumstances under which the physician may well be justified in offering different advice. In maternity work there are usually several good ways of attaining the same end and while one physician may favor one method, another may prefer a quite different approach. What follows, therefore, is not fixed, but must be considered as subject to revision at any time by your physician — whose word should be final because he knows your individual case.

Do not hesitate to bring to your physician any question that may be bothering you. Above all, ask *him* your questions, *not* your friends at the bridge table. Just as some people enjoy talking about their surgical operations, so certain women seem to enjoy expatiating upon their experiences in childbirth, and, of course, in order to make the story a good one, a little exaggeration now and then is common practice. This "bridge-table obstetrics" is usually based on two or three personal experiences at the most — related ordinarily with more gusto than accuracy — plus stray bits of garbled information assembled from one place and another. Here the expectant mother may receive all kinds of gratuitous advice with a sprinkling of taboos and old superstitions thrown in for good measure; she will hear this good doctor and that good doctor misquoted until neither physician would recognize his original statement; and she may even listen to tales of woe and disaster from dour calamity-mongers, to whom this field is particularly dear. All this would be very ludicrous were it not for the fact that many expectant mothers, after such a session, are left in a state of bewilderment, even of fear. Now, under these circumstances, there are two things to do. In the first place, try to understand, as doctors understand, how ridiculous this hodge-podge of misinformation is. If you have the slightest trace of humor in you, now is the time to make the most of it; for this "bridge-table obstetrics" deserves only one thing, a good laugh. And in the second place, if you still have your misgivings, confide them to your doctor. He will tell you the truth, based on thousands of maternity cases, and if you only know the truth, you can have no cause for concern. Again, get your advice from your doctor, not from your friends.

DIET IN PREGNANCY

The old saying that a pregnant woman must eat for two is one of those half truths which has done far more harm than good. The fallacy of the epigram lies in the fact that it implies the necessity for a great increase in the *quantity* of food eaten. This is quite wrong and if heeded not only will result in appalling accretions of fat (which may never be lost), but may even eventuate in certain complications. If viewed from the standpoint of the *quality* of the diet, the old saying has much to recommend it since the foods eaten in pregnancy not only must meet the requirements of the mother's tissues but must include a wide variety of food elements (particularly proteins, minerals and vitamins) which are necessary for the building of the baby's body.

Quantity of Food. — The amount of food consumed by the pregnant woman should be no more and no less than she has been accustomed to eat when not pregnant, for there is no reason to believe that any appreciable increase in the total quantity of food is necessary in pregnancy. To be sure, the growing fetus and enlarging uterus represent an additional amount of tissue to be nourished but this is probably counterbalanced by the reduction in muscular activity which advancing pregnancy entails. You will recall that food values are expressed in "calories," that is, in heat units which indicate the amount of energy which a given food furnishes as it is burned in the body. The Food and Nutrition Board of the National Research Council recommends 2500 calories as the daily allowance for a pregnant woman, the same allowance which it specifies for a moderately active nonpregnant woman.

During the early months of pregnancy the appetite is likely to be poor and in some instances there is an actual distaste for food. When nausea militates still further against adequate food intake there is no little danger of dietary deficiencies developing at this time. As will be discussed in detail when we consider the whole problem of nausea, every effort should be made to work out some form of dietary regime during this period which will supply the important food essentials even though the total quantity of food eaten is temporarily minimal. After the third month the appetite usually increases and sometimes becomes voracious, a source of some annoyance to the young woman who wishes to retain her youthful figure — and what young woman does not? While many subterfuges have been recommended to meet this situation, a certain degree of self-restraint is an essential ingredient in most of them and must be cultivated in some way, at least to the extent of eating only three meals a day and meanwhile avoiding pantry, refrigerator, soda fountain and afternoon teas. Fatty foods and sweets should be especially singled out for curtailment. At meals, of course, there is no reasonable limit to the amount of lettuce, tomatoes, celery, string beans, carrots, beets and asparagus which may be eaten, and by increasing the quantity of such foods to several times the amount ordinarily taken, it is usually possible to maintain a comfortable fullness without gaining abnormally in weight.

On the other hand, attempts to reduce food intake to exceedingly low levels for the purpose of limiting the size of the baby and so facilitating birth are dangerous as well as futile. Although such a practice was advanced some fifty years ago, subsequent investigation has shown that the amount of food taken by the mother has little influence on the size of the child. In general, such reducing diets have no place in the hygiene of the normal pregnant woman, but in case she is markedly overweight or gaining very rapidly, some type of low caloric dietary may be prescribed by the physician in an effort to minimize weight gain. For the benefit of such patients the whole problem of weight control in pregnancy will be discussed in detail in the next chapter.

If you have been accustomed to a varied diet, rich in natural foods such as milk, eggs, fruits and green vegetables, little if any alteration is needed during pregnancy. You should review, nevertheless, the following seven food groups to make certain that each is represented in your dietary each day.

THE BASIC SEVEN FOOD GROUPS [1]

Milk is Nature's most perfect food and is invaluable to the pregnant woman for a number of reasons. In the first place, it contains all the different kinds of mineral elements which are needed by the fetal skeleton. For instance, its high content of calcium (lime) and phosphorus makes it almost indispensable for good growth of bone and teeth; it provides these minerals, moreover, in just

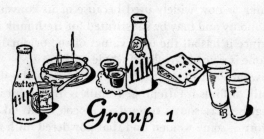

Group 1

Milk and Milk Products
(*One quart daily*)

the correct proportions and in a digestible form which permits their complete utilization by both mother and child. Secondly, it is an excellent source of protein, or tissue-building material. The particular proteins present

---

[1] These seven food groups are essentially the same as those recommended by the National Food Guide, Department of Agriculture, but the order in which they are listed has been changed to give more emphasis to the especial needs of pregnancy.

in milk not only are unexcelled in their ability to promote tissue growth but are the most readily digested
and easily absorbed of all food proteins. Finally, milk
contains some of all of the vitamins, particularly vitamin
A, and safeguards the development of the fetus.

In view of these facts, one quart of milk daily should
be put at the top of your dietary list. At least two glasses
of milk a day should be drunk as such and if desired the
remainder of the quart may be taken in such forms as
cocoa, milk soups, custards and with cereals. Evaporated
milk, which is pure cow's milk minus about one half of
the water, is now widely used because of its convenience
and economy and may be substituted for fresh milk if you
wish, since it has all the food values of the original milk.
The same is true of powdered whole milk.

But what shall we say to the young woman who doesn't
like milk or finds it fattening? If milk is distasteful it may
be disguised as soup, custard or cocoa, and taken in
these forms; some women find that powdered milk mixed
with other foods meets the difficulty. The various forms
of calcium available in medicinal tablets might seem offhand a satisfactory substitute for the calcium of milk.
Although this is doubtless true of some of these products,
the calcium so compounded has been known in some
instances to pass through the intestines unchanged; in
other words, calcium taken in tablet form may not be
absorbed and cannot be regarded, therefore, as an ab-
solutely dependable substitute for that in milk. From a
theoretical standpoint the only acceptable substitute for
milk is cheese, which contains in concentrated form all

the important food elements of milk with the exception of milk sugar. Because it is such a concentrated food, however, it must be eaten with restraint. One ounce of yellow American cheese (a cube about an inch and a quarter in diameter) contains approximately the same amount of calcium, phosphorus, proteins and vitamins as a glass of whole milk (half a pint). Cottage cheese, although rich in protein, is not a satisfactory substitute in respect to calcium, for it would require some five tablespoonfuls to yield the calcium present in half a glass of milk. Used sparingly, let us say an ounce or two a day, American cheese may be used to replace a portion of the milk recommended.

Concerning the fattening effects of milk, it must be recalled that weight gain is simply the result of eating more food than is needed, that is, consuming more calories than the energy requirements call for. As we have said, a quart of milk furnishes barely a third of these requirements and if taken without other foods would certainly result in a decided loss in weight. If gain is excessive, then, it is not the milk which is at fault, but the superimposed foods such as bread, potatoes and desserts. Milk, not these starches and sweets, should be the basic food in pregnancy, for no other can serve so well as the foundation of a complete diet.

As rich sources of vitamin A, iron and other important vitamins and minerals, the green and yellow vegetables stand second in the list of food necessities for the pregnant woman, especially the crisp green vegetables. This food group includes, you recall:

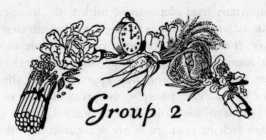

Group 2

Leafy Green and Yellow Vegetables

(*One or more servings daily*)

Asparagus, green	Endive, green
Beans, Lima	Escarole
Beans, snap, green	*Kale
*Broccoli	Lettuce, leaf
Brussels sprouts	*Mustard greens
Cabbage, green	Okra
*Chard	Peas, green
*Collards	Peppers, green and red
*Spinach	Carrots
*Turnip greens	Pumpkins
*Wild greens	Squash, winter yellow
Other greens, including	Sweet potatoes
salad greens	

The items starred are particularly high in iron and vitamin content and should be given preference whenever possible.

The cooking should be brief and a minimum of water used. Since prolonged heating is likely to destroy vitamin content, ten to fifteen minutes in boiling water should be the limit for most of the vegetables mentioned and in some instances much less. The water may be saved and used as a stock for soups, if desired, since it contains valuable minerals and vitamins extracted from the vegetable. Canned or frozen vegetables may be used in the place of fresh if desired; the vitamin content is often higher than that of vegetables cooked at home.

In addition to their value as nutrient agents, these vegetables deserve an important place in the diet of the pregnant woman as laxative agents since their fibrous framework increases the bulk of the bowel content and thereby stimulates the muscular, eliminative action of the intestines.

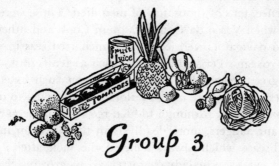

Group 3

Citrus Fruit, Tomatoes, Raw Cabbage, Etc.

(Two or more servings daily)

Grapefruit	Cabbage, raw
Grapefruit juice	Greens, salad
Kumquats	Peppers, green, raw
Lemons	Turnips, raw
Limes	

Orange juice	A large serving of the
Oranges	above vegetables can
Tangerines	be substituted for the
	fruits listed in this
Tomatoes	group.
Tomato juice	
	If foods in Group 3 are
Cantaloupes (musk-	hard to get, use more,
melons)	especially raw, from
Pineapples, raw	Groups 2 and 6.
Strawberries, raw	

Less than a century and a half ago the importance of fresh fruit in the diet was not appreciated and, as a consequence, tens of thousands of men died. Those were the days when Vasco da Gama, Captain Cook and other intrepid navigators were exploring uncharted seas in year-long voyages. Perishable goods, such as fruit, milk, eggs and green vegetables, had no place on such extended cruises, and the fare of the sailors was restricted to dried and salty foods. Although hidden reefs and icebergs were constant dangers, more deadly than these was an insidious disease which always afflicted the men after a few months at sea, a malady characterized by growing listlessness, bone pains, and swollen, bleeding gums. The disease became known as scurvy. The ravages of scurvy were such that three quarters of a ship's crew often succumbed; but not until the eighteenth century was its cause finally discovered: absence of fruit. In 1854 a law was passed in England requiring that fruit juice be rationed out daily on long voyages, and it was because of this dole of lemon juice that English sailors began to be called "limeys." Here, also, is the genesis of "Limehouse" — the water-front district in London where the fruit was stored.

We now know that these sailors died because a certain substance necessary for life was absent from their diet; this substance is found only in fresh foods, particularly fruits, and is now called vitamin C. We might mention other dire and fatal diseases which result when certain other vitamins are withheld completely; but today we seldom see examples of complete vitamin deprivation. We do see, however, many cases of partial vitamin defi-ciency, and these are particularly insidious because less readily recognized. Lowered resistance to infection, boils, bleeding gums, defective teeth, dry and blotchy skin, acne, loss of hair and brittle fingernails are some of the com-moner disorders which result from partial vitamin lack.

Fruits, particularly oranges, lemons and grapefruit, are not only rich sources of vitamin C, but contain liberal amounts of other important vitamins. From a nutritional standpoint tomatoes fall into this same group and may be substituted for fruits as desired. Another excellent and in-expensive source of vitamin C is raw cabbage, which may be introduced as slaw into many an appetizing salad com-bination. Other raw fruits may be advantageously added to this salad bowl and no end of healthful dishes with unsurpassed flavors devised. Peaches, plums, pineapples and apricots are but a few of the fruits which may be combined with lettuce, water cress, slaw, etc., to yield vitamin-rich, health-giving dishes. The noted beauty au-thority, Mme. Helena Rubinstein, stresses again and again in her writings the fact that beauty is not merely "skin deep" but depends on vibrant internal health; clear skin, glistening hair, and all that goes with the glamor and vitality of youth, she points out, are to be found *par excellence* in a diet rich in raw fruits and vegetables. During pregnancy, when the need for vitamins and minerals is greatly increased, these raw foods become doubly necessary.

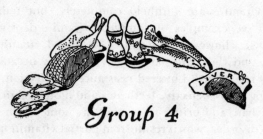

Group 4

Meat, Poultry, Fish and Eggs
(*One or more servings daily*)

One egg, better two, should be included in the menu each day since the yolks, in particular, are rich sources of iron, vitamins and tissue-building proteins. Since we are again stressing the desirability of an iron-containing food in the dietary of the pregnant woman, it may be well to explain the reason. The function of iron in the body is exceedingly important, for it is an essential element in the oxygen-carrying material of the red blood cells, hemoglobin. This is the substance which makes blood red and gives to cheeks their ruddiness, and when we say that a person is pale or anemic-looking, we mean to imply that his blood is low in this iron-containing pigment, hemoglobin. Despite the importance of iron, the amount present in the body is small, about a tenth of an ounce in a full-grown healthy person. Moreover, it appears impossible for the adult body to store iron for future use; this means that there is no reserve supply to draw on and that the iron needs must be met day by day in the diet. Now, throughout the latter part of pregnancy the fetus, unlike the adult, stores iron in its liver for future use; this is wise foresight on the part of the fetus because he will have to subsist after birth largely on milk, which is low in iron, and he will therefore need these reserved stores. Since the fetus also requires iron for building his own red cells, the demand imposed on the mother for this mineral is so great that about a third of pregnant women develop some degree of anemia through lack of it. The necessity for ample amounts of iron-containing foods in pregnancy, therefore, cannot be overemphasized. While the iron supplied by one egg represents only one tenth of the total daily need, this form of iron is assimilated by the body with particular ease and should not be neglected.

Although meat was formerly regarded as harmful to the expectant mother there is increasing reason to believe that moderate amounts are not only permissible but necessary. It is my own custom to recommend one serving of lean meat daily and to suggest that liver be eaten once weekly, at least. Liver differs considerably in its nutritive values from the muscle tissue so generally preferred by Americans. It is not only exceedingly rich in iron and in copper, which is necessary for the utilization of iron, but furnishes certain essential substances needed for the building of red blood cells; at the same time it is abundantly supplied with important vitamins. The amount of liver eaten at one time need not be large; for instance, one small piece, three inches square and one half inch thick, contains more iron than two eggs. Oysters are excelled only by liver as a source of blood-building materials and may be substituted for liver during the winter months.

Because of the tendency to develop anemia in pregnancy and the difficulty of meeting iron needs by natural foods, many physicians make it a routine to prescribe an iron compound in the form of capsules or tablets for daily ingestion. Various vitamins are often included in the capsule.

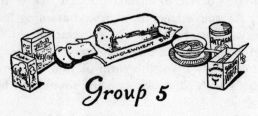

Group 5

Whole-Wheat Bread and Cereals
(*Every day*)

Breads:
  Whole-wheat
  Dark rye
  Enriched
  Rolls or biscuits made
    with whole-wheat or
    enriched flour

Corn meal, whole-grain
  or enriched

Grits, enriched

Cereals:
  Whole-wheat

Oatmeal bread

Crackers, enriched,
    whole-grain, soya

Flour, enriched whole-
wheat, other whole-
grain

Rolled oats
Brown rice
Converted rice
Other cereals, if whole-
    grain or restored

Prior to 1830 wheat flour was obtained simply by grind-
ing the whole grain between stones. As a result the
bread eaten in those days contained both the germ and
the outer shell (bran) of the wheat kernel. It was brown
in color, naturally, and somewhat coarser in texture than
the bread we eat today, but it was so nutritious and
health-building that our ancestors, you remember, called
it the "staff of life." The invention of the roller mill for
the manufacture of wheat flour, about 1830, appeared to
mark a great advance. By eliminating the germ and the
shell, it made possible the production of flour that was
less subject to deterioration than whole-wheat and consequently more suitable for commerce; the flour, moreover, was white in color and fine in consistency, qualities
which not only appealed to the eye but suggested greater
purity. The new process was a sweeping commercial success and today white bread is the most important staple
of the American dietary.

During recent years, physicians have suffered a rude
awakening in learning that these modern refinements in
milling have deprived bread of some of its most important nutritive constituents. Both the germ and the shell

of the wheat kernel are rich in iron, protein and two essential vitamins, the B vitamins and vitamin E. Deficiency in certain of the B vitamins reveals itself principally by inflammation and degeneration of the nerves; in its absence heaviness of the legs and tenderness in the calf muscles ensue, while ability to walk even short distances is impaired; digestive disturbances are also common, particularly loss of appetite and nausea. From the viewpoint of the expectant mother, however, it is even more important to know that both the B vitamins and vitamin E are indispensable for successful childbearing. Experiments in the lower animals show that if either of these vitamins is completely withheld during the first half of pregnancy, something like a miscarriage invariably follows; while if they are omitted during the second half, the offspring are likely to be sickly. Also, studies on human beings indicate that during pregnancy more of the B vitamins are required to saturate the body than are needed in the nonpregnant state.

It has been estimated that modern milling methods do away with more than 90 per cent of the B vitamins present in the old stone-ground flour. An almost ludicrous example of the inadequacy of modern diets in this respect was recently cited in England. A study was made of the foods which the city of London utilized a century ago, in feeding paupers and prisoners; these foods with their quantities are all specified in the Poor Law of London and hence it has been possible to calculate the nutritive value of these old rations and compare them with modern menus. The startling fact was discovered that the food which was penuriously doled out to these indigent in 1838 contained twice as much of the B vitamins as was present in the dietaries of the highest income groups of London in 1937. Conditions in the United States are doubtless similar and the conclusion seems inescapable that a large fraction of our population subsists on diets of borderline adequacy in respect to the B vitamins.

If American dietaries as a whole are unsatisfactory in this regard, as physicians and nutritionists now believe, they are particularly inadequate to meet the increased needs during pregnancy. Accordingly, whole-wheat bread should replace white bread in your dietary to the extent, let us say, of two or three slices a day. In addition, opportunity should be seized at breakfast to eat still more whole-grain products in the form of rolled oats, shredded-wheat biscuit, puffed wheat and other brown cereals.

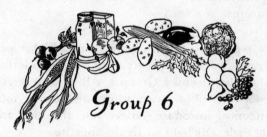

Group 6

Potatoes and Other Vegetables and Fruits

(*Two or more servings daily*)

Potatoes	Apples
Sweet potatoes	Apricots
	Avocados
Artichokes	Bananas
Beets	Berries

Cabbage, white
Cauliflower
Celery
Corn, sweet
Cucumbers
Eggplant
Leeks
Lettuce, head
Mushrooms
Onions
Parsnips
Radishes
Rutabagas
Salsify, or oyster plant
Sauerkraut
Squash, summer
Turnips

Cherries
Cranberries
Currants
Dates
Figs
Grapes
Peaches
Pears
Persimmons
Pineapple, canned
Pineapple juice, canned
Plums
Prunes
Raisins
Rhubarb
Watermelons

Most vegetables in this class contain a higher percentage of carbohydrate and hence yield a higher caloric value than those listed under Group 2. All of these vegetables and fruits contribute worthwhile amounts of minerals and vitamins, introduce variety into the diet, and because of their bulk help satisfy the appetite.

As an essential food, butter is the least important of the Basic 7. It is true that it is very rich in vitamin A but this vitamin is amply supplied by several of the other food groups mentioned. It is nevertheless included because of the taste it gives to certain foods which are essential; for instance, most people find a slice of bread rather unappealing without butter. If excessive weight

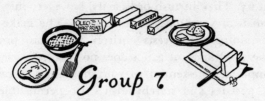

Group 7

Butter and Fortified Margarine

gain is a problem, however, it must be partaken of sparingly because of its well-known fattening propensities.

* * * *

To summarize, then, you should include in your menu each day one or more items from each of the following food groups:

1. Milk (one quart).
2. Leafy green and yellow vegetables (one or more servings).
3. Citrus fruit, tomatoes, raw cabbage, etc. (two or more servings).
4. Meat, poultry, fish and eggs (one egg; better two; lean meat, one or more servings; liver, once or more weekly, if possible).
5. Whole-wheat bread and cereals (two or more servings).
6. Potatoes and other vegetables and fruits (two or more servings).
7. Butter and fortified margarine (a small amount).

The above are basic, protective foods designed to safeguard you and your baby, and should be regarded as obligatory. They furnish ordinarily, however, only about two thirds of your daily requirements. The make-up of the remaining third rests entirely with you, provided that the total amount eaten does not exceed your usual consumption. If essential to your happiness, occasional sweets, pastries and starchy dishes are permissible; but unless you aspire to a whole flight of double chins, partake of these sparingly and watch the scales!

Cod-Liver Oil. — There remains another extremely important vitamin to be considered, vitamin D. Without this vitamin the body is unable to change calcium and phosphorus into bone; it is hence essential for normal bone formation, for the normal development of teeth and for the maintenance of sound tooth structure. Having already stressed the needs of the growing fetus for calcium, it is scarcely necessary to add that in pregnancy adequate amounts of vitamin D are imperative. But vitamin D is peculiar among vitamins in that it is formed naturally in the body as the result of exposure to the sun's rays; we may say accordingly that one rich source of this vitamin is sunshine. Another, of course, is cod-liver oil. It follows, then, that the amount of cod-liver oil needed by the pregnant woman depends on the degree to which she is exposed to the sun's rays. In climates without much sunshine, particularly during the latter six months of pregnancy when the baby's teeth are being formed, cod-liver oil is a valuable safeguard. On the other hand, if liberal exposure to sunshine is possible and feasible to the extent that a slight tan on the legs, arms and back can be maintained, it may be unnecessary. Since the latter circumstance is rarely attainable the year around, it is customary for many physicians to recommend vitamin D daily, particularly during the winter months. Physicians hold differing views about this, however, and the opinion of your own medical attendant should be sought and followed. If you find even small amounts of cod-liver oil objectionable, he will doubtless be able to suggest some more palatable substitute. Under no circumstances, however, attempt to doctor yourself with any of the concentrated vitamin D products, such as viosterol, without your physician's advice and instructions.

Iodine. — Although only infinitesimal quantities of iodine are needed by the body, a small amount is necessary for the health of mother and baby alike. This may be ensured by eating sea food twice a week or by the use of iodized salt. In certain localities in the United States, notably around the Great Lakes and in the Northwest, the water and soil have lost their iodine and consequently the foods grown in these regions may provide inadequate amounts. Not infrequently doctors in these localities prescribe small amounts of iodine for expectant mothers, but iodine should only be taken upon the advice and under the immediate supervision of a physician.

Foods to Avoid. — It is only common sense to avoid any article of diet which you know disagrees with you. During pregnancy the stomach and other digestive organs are encroached upon by the growing uterus and will often not tolerate foods which ordinarily cause no difficulty. Experience shows that the following articles of diet are common offenders: rich foods and condiments of all sorts, fried foods, sausage, smoked or salt fish and rich pastries. You may even find that some of the foods recommended under "Leafy green and yellow vegetables" may at first prove upsetting. If so, it very probably means that the digestive tract has become so pampered by artificially prepared foods, which feel gentle and velvety, that at the outset it is unable to stand foods in their natural state. Under such circumstances there is no time so good as the present to swing over to correct eating habits. This must be done gradually, however, increasing little by little the amount of raw foods taken, remembering always that their digestibility is immeasurably increased by prolonged chewing.

If there is any one substance which should be curtailed during pregnancy, it is salt. In the first place, the amount of salt consumed by the average person is far in excess of human requirements. Second, even if *no* salt were added to foods either in the kitchen or at the table, this mineral is so widely distributed in food materials that the likelihood of shortage would be exceedingly remote. Finally, there is a definite relationship between the amount of salt eaten and the amount of water retained by the body; that is, the greater the salt intake the greater the tendency of tissues to absorb water. The tissues of the pregnant woman manifest a particular avidity for water, as is evidenced by the tendency of the face and fingers to become puffy, and if, superimposed on this tendency, there is an excess of salt in the diet, the tissues may become actually waterlogged with dire consequences. It is a good rule to add no salt to the food at the table, and in the kitchen to add a little less than you would like.

Fluids. — Six glasses of water should be drunk daily

and more in hot weather. An ample fluid intake in pregnancy seems to flush out the kidneys and prevent certain disturbances of these organs not uncommon at this time. Tea and coffee may be drunk as usual provided the former is not found constipating or the latter sleep-disturbing.

Small amounts of alcohol, let us say a cocktail now and then or a glass of wine, are harmless, but may prove a nuisance in aggravating frequency of urination.

Gain in Weight. — During the first three and a half months of pregnancy the weight is usually stationary and may show a slight loss. During the latter two thirds of the process, however, there is a steady gain, over some twenty-four weeks, which averages about a pound a week. The greater part of this twenty-four-pound increment is quite understandable, as shown by the following figures:

Baby	7	pounds
Afterbirth	1	pound
Amniotic fluid	1½	pounds
Increase in weight of uterus	2	pounds
Increase in blood	1	pound
Increase in weight of breasts	1½	pounds
	14	pounds

The remaining ten pounds represent in part general accumulation of fat and in part the increased amount of fluid which tissues tend to retain at this time. Gains between twenty and twenty-four pounds are natural and in keeping with good health; they are usually lost, moreover, after the baby is born. On the contrary, increases in weight of thirty pounds and more are undesirable for a number of reasons. In the first place, they represent unnecessary poundage for the muscles of the legs and back to carry about and this suddenly imposed strain is a common cause of backache and pain in the legs. Certainly, you will feel much better if you keep your weight gain in the neighborhood of twenty pounds. Second, not a few complications of pregnancy and labor are associated with excessive increments in weight. In other words, you and your baby will be healthier and safer if you follow this advice. Finally, these huge accretions of fat are likely to be permanent acquisitions which can be removed only by the most rigorous dieting. Your appearance, then, will be everlastingly better if you adhere to the rule of keeping weight gain near twenty pounds.

GENERAL HYGIENE IN PREGNANCY

Clothing. — The most important consideration in regard to the expectant mother's wardrobe is that it should be attractive. This may sound like a superficial observation but it is profoundly true. Yes, more important than knowing the dangers of circular garters and high heels is the knowledge that you are well-groomed, because only then (if you are like most women) will you really enjoy entertaining your friends and meeting your husband's friends, and in turn visiting their homes. Pregnancy is no time to be a recluse. The more you are in the company of others, the better off you are; indeed, I have long chronicled the impression that patients who start in labor while playing bridge invariably have an easy time.

This is simply another way of saying that the woman who cultivates a certain oblivion to the fact that she is pregnant (although obeying the ordinary rules of diet and hygiene) does much better than her introspective sister.

As the appearance of many expectant mothers attests, it is possible to look attractive at this time as at any other. To be sure, the abdominal rotundity is a handicap, but, for some reason, during the middle months of pregnancy women develop a special radiance which is most becoming and tends to offset this. Moreover, maternity dresses are so ingeniously contrived these days that they resemble an optical illusion in their ability to beguile the eye in regard to your real contour — which, incidentally, is always more noticeable to you than to anyone else. Patterns for such garments, as well as the ready-made dresses themselves, are readily and inexpensively obtained at any department store and it is a good idea to exercise your ingenuity on this problem.

From the standpoint of your physical well-being there are only a few precautions to be kept in mind. Naturally, whatever you wear should keep you comfortably warm. Since American homes are kept at a rather high temperature, the wearing of heavy underclothes when indoors is unnecessary. However, when out of doors on cold or wet days, every care should be taken to prevent chilling by wearing a warm coat, sweater, overshoes and possibly heavier underclothing. With the obliteration of the waistline by the growing uterus about the fifth month, it becomes increasingly difficult (and increasingly undesirable) to hang clothes from the hips and, in so far as is possible, they should be suspended from the shoulders. Constriction of the abdomen by tight bands interferes with your breathing, impedes free movement of the baby and may even have an injurious effect on the uterus. For these reasons, as well as for the sake of your appearance, all clothes should be full and flowing.

In regard to outer garments, attractive maternity skirts are available which have an expandable waistband. This can be adjusted to a level just above the uterus, sparing any pressure on that organ. In combination with an appealing maternity blouse, this is a justly popular costume.

Garters. — Since the growing uterus not only bulges forward but presses backward against the veins which drain blood from the legs, the circulation in the lower extremities is often sluggish in pregnancy. Herein lies the common reason for swelling of the ankles so commonly seen during the later weeks. Tight circular garters and rolled stockings obstruct still further the return flow of blood from the legs and predispose to varicose veins. Suspensory garters should therefore be worn instead, being hung either from a garter belt or from a maternity corset.

Shoes. — There are two undeniable reasons why expectant mothers should wear low, broad heels, but women who have long been accustomed to high heels sometimes find this change so discomforting and awkward that a compromise is often necessary. The objections to high heels are obvious enough. In the first place, from the standpoint of weight distribution, the pregnant woman is not unlike a person carrying a twelve-pound basket pressed against the abdomen. In order to support the weight and maintain equilibrium, it is necessary to tilt the torso backward. The resultant "sway-back" posture puts additional strain on the muscles of the abdomen, back and thighs and accounts for many of the muscular aches which sometimes accompany the later weeks. Since high heels accentuate the "sway-back" posture, they may cause, or aggravate, muscular cramps in these regions as pregnancy progresses. The second objection to high heels is their tendency to cause accidents both in the form of tripping on stairs and of turning the ankle. In view of these facts, excessively high heels are certainly to be avoided. A satisfactory compromise is a heel in the neighborhood of one and a half inches high which is broad enough to support your increased weight without danger of turning. Since there is a slight tendency for the feet to swell in the evenings as pregnancy advances, it is well to purchase shoes a trifle larger than usual.

Maternity Corset. — The chief purpose of a maternity corset is to promote your comfort during the latter months of pregnancy. In women who have never worn a corset, it is usually unnecessary and may even prove a hindrance rather than a help to comfort, particularly in warm weather. A number of expectant mothers, however, find them a distinct aid after the fifth month, particularly women who have had previous children. The function of such a corset is several-fold. In the first place, it supports the growing uterus from below upward without compressing it and without exerting pressure on the upper abdomen, thus allowing ample room for deep breathing and for the baby's activity; in this way it takes over the work of the lower abdominal muscles in supporting the uterus and thereby rests them. Second, it provides a stay for the back and in this way relieves the back muscles of a certain amount of strain. Finally, by fitting snugly around the pelvic girdle, it holds the bones of the pelvis tightly together and tends to correct a certain "wobbliness" which develops in this structure as pregnancy advances.

In choosing a maternity corset, several considerations should be borne in mind. Since it should be put on lying down, a type with hooks or a zipper in front is most convenient. In the lying posture the uterus naturally falls backward into its most inconspicuous and natural position and if the corset is applied under these circumstances, the support it gives not only is greater but is more evenly distributed. This is readily demonstrated as follows: Put the garment on in the standing position and tighten the lacings on the sides and back, from below upward to such an extent that the corset is rather too snug for comfort. Now loosen the front, lie down, raise the hips slightly and close the front from below upward, and it will be found that the corset is altogether comfortable. Although many maternity corsets have elastic inserts, these lose their supportive power very rapidly, and consequently corsets of nonelastic material such as brocade or damask are ordinarily preferable. It is needless to add that the corset should be fitted by a competent person and a type chosen which is in keeping with your size and build.

During the first half of pregnancy, an elastic girdle or panty girdle, without stays, may contribute to your comfort, especially if you have been accustomed to wearing one. But it is not necessary.

Brassière. — The breasts are much more comfortable when supported by a brassière of the uplift or sling type which lifts each breast upward and inward toward the opposite shoulder. Brassières which flatten the breasts are injurious and should never be worn.

Bathing. — During the last six weeks tub baths should give way to daily sponge baths or showers. Among other good reasons for this, the equilibrium is likely to be uncertain at this time and there is danger of losing one's foothold on the slippery tub and falling against its side. Throughout pregnancy long "soaks" in a very hot bath are to be avoided since they are more likely to cause fatigue than comfort and tend to produce an undesirable congestion in the pelvis.

Teeth. — The old saying, "For every child a tooth," is based upon the belief that the fetus takes calcium from the mother's teeth. Although modern investigation refutes this contention, there is no doubt that some women do suffer markedly from dental decay during pregnancy. Accordingly, the dentist should be consulted early and his recommendations followed. The old notion that dental work causes miscarriage is without basis. On the contrary, a thorough overhauling of the teeth is a good preventive measure against this and other accidents of pregnancy; extractions are preferably done under local anesthesia. Meanwhile assiduous care should be used in cleansing the teeth after meals and in the use of an alkaline mouthwash night and morning.

Nipples. — As we have already noted, there is a tendency for the colostrum, the sticky fluid which the breasts secrete in pregnancy, to cake on the nipples and cause irritation. To remove this, the nipples should be gently cleansed at the time of the bath with a soft cloth, warm water and soap. This may be done as often as is necessary, particular care being used to dry the nipples thoroughly afterward.

In regard to further care of the nipples in pregnancy, medical opinion varies so widely as to be altogether inconsistent. Some physicians recommend alcohol to harden the nipples, others oil to soften them, while many consider it preferable to do nothing at all. The objective, of course, is so to prepare the nipples that cracks and little tender spots will not develop when the baby nurses. It is possibly the consensus that somewhat better results are obtained if the nipples are anointed with cocoa butter every evening during the last two months. However, it is advisable that your own doctor give you instructions about this after he has inspected your nipples.

Douches. — Douches should not be taken in pregnancy without specific instructions from your doctor.

Sexual Intercourse. — Under no circumstances is sexual intercourse permissible during the last month of pregnancy. This is one rule which is extremely important and absolute. Prior to the last month of pregnancy intercourse is harmless in moderation.

Bowels. — The bowels should move once daily, better twice. If they do not, immediate and intelligent measures should be instituted to correct the difficulty, which is an extremely common one in pregnancy. The treatment of constipation is considered in detail on pages 103-104.

Exercise. — Regular exercise in the open air, even though it be no more than a half hour's stroll to a friend's house, should form part of your daily routine. For everyone, probably, walking is the best type of exercise; for the pregnant woman there can be no question of its superiority. It stimulates the eliminative activity of the lungs, skin and bowels, keeps the muscles in good condition and promotes sleep — to say nothing of the fact that it takes you away from house and self and thereby fosters other interests. The amount of exercise which the expectant mother can comfortably and safely carry out, however, is so related to what she has been accustomed to that it is difficult, as well as undesirable, to lay down any hard and fast rules. For the average woman a mile or so a day is about the right amount, but it is advisable to divide this into several short walks rather than to push oneself to the point of fatigue merely to cover a definite distance. Better inertia than any form of activity pushed grimly to the point of fatigue. Gardening, if you are so fortunate as to have a garden, is an ideal form of exercise. Light housework, although in no way a substitute for out-of-door exercise, is a helpful form of activity and may be continued with profit throughout pregnancy; it should be stopped short of fatigue, however, and in no event should include the lifting of heavy objects.

Violent activity is to be avoided, particularly anything which involves jolting, sudden motion or running. Although physicians vary widely in the forms of exercises they permit in pregnancy, they usually disapprove of horseback riding, tennis and skating — not so much by reason of the sports themselves as because of the attendant danger of falling. Golf is usually permissible if played leisurely and limited to nine holes. If you are accustomed to swimming there is ordinarily no objection to this sport during the first half of pregnancy provided the water is reasonably warm and diving is omitted. Dancing is harmless, as a rule, if indulged in moderately. However, not a few experienced physicians hold different views in regard to these three diversions — golf, swimming and dancing — and it would be well to ascertain the opinion of your own doctor concerning them.

Automobile Trips. — Anyone who has ridden three hundred miles a day in an automobile knows that the experience is fatiguing, no matter how good the roads. Since pregnant women are prone to tire easily, common sense dictates that prolonged automobile trips should be planned conservatively and your doctor's approval obtained. Restriction of travel to short trips was the rule for expectant mothers prior to World War II, when many women found it necessary to follow their husbands regardless of distance or modes of conveyance. It is now possible to apply data compiled during that era to show that travel, almost regardless of distance and type of conveyance, has little or no harmful effect on pregnancy. Nevertheless, because of its tiring effects, automobile travel should be interspersed by rest periods of 10 to 15 minutes every 100 miles or so; and 300 miles a day should be the uppermost limit.

As for driving a car yourself, it would be best to inquire of your own physician. It is usually permitted during the first six months of pregnancy, at least, if reasonable care is exercised in regard to speed and accident.

Travel. — For traveling distances greater than three hundred miles, the railway is the safest as well as the most comfortable vehicle. Ocean voyages are without objection provided there is no tendency to nausea and proper care is taken to avoid injury in rough weather.

Air travel, whether in jet or propeller planes, is likewise safe. *However,* during the last month of pregnancy (and in the case of one airline, during the last two months), the expectant mother must present to the airline a certificate from her physician, dated within 72 hours of departure, attesting that she is in good physical condition and stating the expected date of confinement.

Travel late in pregnancy is unwise for the simple reason that many babies, as we have seen, are born earlier than the calculated date of delivery. It is good rule throughout the last month of pregnancy to be within easy reach of the place set for your confinement.

Moving. — For obvious reasons many expectant parents seize upon pregnancy as an appropriate time to move into larger quarters. Nothing entails so much hard, backbreaking labor as moving. Even though a score of movers are employed, there are few women who can forbear helping with this piece of furniture or that basket of bric-a-brac; moreover, after the movers leave, you are only theoretically "moved," for there is no end of arranging yet to do in the new home; one task leads to another endlessly and often a state of debilitating fatigue results. Pregnancy and moving, then, are incompatible and the latter had best be deferred until the baby is six months old. If you feel, however, that a change of quarters is obligatory, follow a course something as follows: Turn the whole business over to your husband, spend "moving day" at a friend's house resting, and go to your new home only after your husband (with the help of available relatives, perhaps) has the place in proper order. Your welfare and that of your baby demand that you act a complete invalid on such an occasion.

Employment. — The expectant mother who is employed will naturally want to know how late in pregnancy she may continue her work and how early she may return after the baby is born. Clerical work may be kept up as long as desired. Work which involves much in the way of physical activity or entails long hours of standing should be stopped two months before the expected day of confinement. Although employers nowadays are very liberal-minded about such matters, there are naturally certain positions which cannot be held after the pregnancy becomes apparent. If this is a factor, plans should be made to discontinue work before the end of the fifth month. Following delivery, six weeks are needed for the reproductive organs to return to normal, for the mother to regain her full strength and for the baby to get a good start. Accordingly, no commitments should be made about returning to work until the baby is from six to eight weeks old.

Rest. — During the early months of pregnancy many women experience an almost uncontrollable desire to sleep, a good hint that more rest is required at this time. In addition to the usual amount of sleep at night, let us say eight or ten hours, it is highly desirable that the expectant mother lie down for an hour every afternoon with shoes off and clothes loosened. If she sleeps, well and good; if not, she will still feel refreshed after such an hour of complete relaxation. During the last few weeks a similar rest should be taken in the morning.

Smoking. — Current interest in the harmful effects of cigarette smoking, quite apart from pregnancy, has stirred new concern over the possible bearing of smoking by pregnant women on the well-being of the infant. As the result of extensive studies on the question, it seems clear that the newborn of mothers who smoke tend to weigh slightly less than those of mothers who do not smoke. But whether this lower birth weight indicates an injurious effect has not been established. Regardless of these findings, most physicians recommend that smoking should be curtailed in pregnancy to ten cigarettes or less a day.

Chapter IV

WEIGHT CONTROL IN
PREGNANCY

THE desirability of restricting weight gain in pregnancy was stressed in the previous chapter and a few general measures mentioned by which this end can be attained in most cases. Many expectant mothers, however, gain excessively despite apparent attempts to eliminate rich desserts and snacks between meals, and hence require more specific help in weight curtailment than is afforded by the previous pages. Since this group is a large one and since obstetricians are emphasizing more and more the importance of weight control — some insisting on as little as fifteen pounds' gain — the necessity of considering this problem in some detail is apparent.

If your weight gain after the third month is of the order of one half to three-quarters of a pound a week, that is, at a rate which will not yield a total gain of more than twenty pounds, it may be unnecessary for you to read this chapter. If, however, the scales show a weekly increase in excess of one pound, so that you face a total increment of twenty-five pounds or more, it will repay you to study carefully these next few pages. In addition to the several advantages which you yourself will derive at the present time from better dietary management (as stressed on pages 71-72), there are other even more important benefits to be gained from a general familiarity with this subject. As all life-insurance statistics attest, obesity is a menace to the well-being and longevity of every man and woman; and obesity, with rare exceptions, is the result of faulty dietary habits. Accordingly, the general principles set forth in the Eight Steps in Weight Control described below, although designed for your help in pregnancy, may well be remembered over the years to the advantage of every member of your family.

STEP 1

Acquaint yourself with the amazing fattening potentialities of certain common, nonessential foods — foods which in many people's minds scarcely deserve that term at all because most of them are likely to be regarded as mere snacks without appreciable effect on total caloric intake. Actually, these little extras taken between meals or at bedtime constitute one of the most common causes for excessive weight gain in pregnancy and at other times. Even a glass of ginger ale or a Coca-Cola averages 100 calories. A 5-cent chocolate bar approximates more than 300 calories. A single cocktail or highball runs 200 calories. A doughnut (without icing) plus a cup of cocoa yields 400 calories, while the average malted milk as served at soda fountains contains some 500 calories. Pie à la mode approximates 600 calories. Now, when it is recalled, as stated on page 51, that 2500 calories per day is generally recognized as a satisfactory allowance for pregnancy — really, the uppermost limit — it is plain that these "little snacks" mentioned above loom tremendously large in relationship to the total caloric allotment. And they simply must be eliminated if you are gaining ex-

cessively. When hungry between meals take the glass of
milk scheduled for dinner, omitting it from your evening
meal.

A list of some of the more common nonessential foods,
with the caloric values of average servings, is given in
Table 1 (pages 93-96). If the expectant mother who is
having trouble with the scales will but glance this list
through, she will possibly be surprised that many items
which she scarcely regarded as foods at all contribute an
appalling number of calories; and this indeed may be
her main difficulty. In regard to desserts, Groups 3 and 4
(average servings equal 300 and 400 calories, respectively) should be noted particularly — not overlooking
the fact that the most common dessert of all, pie, falls in
the 400 calorie group. Certainly, all items in these two
groups, as well as other rich creamy desserts, must be
given up if you desire earnestly to curtail weight gain.

STEP 2

Remember that the way in which a food is prepared
may affect its caloric or fattening value almost as much
as the character of the food itself. Failure to heed this
fact has resulted in many women gaining weight on diets
which should cause them, theoretically at least, to lose.
Thus, in a typical day's menu as shown in Table 2
(page 97), the calories may range between 2500 and
3600, depending on the ingredients used in the recipe,
the manner of the cooking, and of course, on the particular type of fruit, meat, dessert, etc., chosen. Perhaps the
simplest example to show how the preparation of a
food affects its caloric value is to be found in fried foods.

Although the caloric content of a poached or boiled egg is about 80 calories and is so calculated in dietary lists, once that egg is fried its caloric value jumps to around 120 calories because of the fat absorbed by the egg in cooking. A level tablespoonful of fat, let it be emphasized, yields approximately 120 calories. Furthermore, nearly all foods which do not contain eggs are dipped in flour or crumbs before frying and this adds greatly to their caloric value. In regard to soups and desserts, it is common knowledge that those made with milk are of much lower caloric content than those made with cream and that those made with skimmed milk are still lower. When flour or cheese in addition to cream is used, as in escalloped or au gratin dishes, the calories soar to unbelievable heights; and in general for this group of foods, the smoother and the more delicious the taste (alas!), the higher the caloric value.

The intrinsic caloric value of foods of the same type varies widely. We have already seen that a dessert may range from 100 to 400 calories and more. Fruits also show considerable variation according to their degree of sweetness. Canned fruit may be very high because of the sugar in the syrup, as noted in Table 1 under "Miscellaneous." Likewise, meats vary greatly in their caloric content, lean meats being low and those with much fat in their substance being high. As an example of the latter, an average serving of linked country sausage may exceed 600 calories.

In summary, Step 2 consists in familiarizing yourself with the relative caloric or fattening values of foods as they are actually prepared and served — and acting thereupon. It is neither necessary nor desirable to memorize caloric values of foods. Just remember (1) that fried foods invariably possess a high caloric content, and must be curtailed or eliminated altogether; (2) that milk, preferably skimmed milk, should be substituted for cream in preparing soups and desserts; and (3) that lean meats rather than fatty meats must be chosen and fresh fruit rather than canned.

STEP 3

Make certain that the size of servings eaten is not excessive and that but one is taken. The standard household measuring cup, as shown (actual size) in Figure 6, is used by dietitians as a sort of reference standard in describing amounts of food. The purpose of reproducing it here is merely to facilitate better visualization of what is meant below by average servings. It is most certainly *not* the intention to suggest any actual measurement of servings.

Average servings of some of the more common foods are considered to be something as follows:

Cereals	¾ to 1 cup
Potatoes or equivalents such as corn, Lima beans, peas, macaroni, etc.	½ cup
Cooked vegetable	½ cup
Butter	1 pat, 1″ x 1″ x ¼″
Desserts such as puddings, custard, ice cream, gelatin desserts, etc.	½ cup

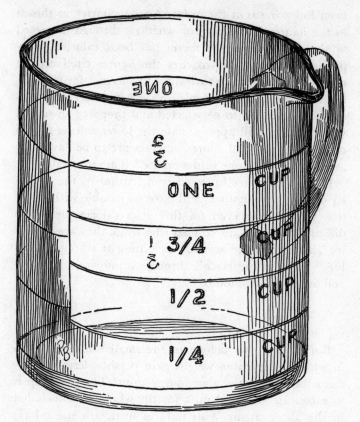

Figure 6. Standard Measuring Cup (Actual Size).

STEP 4

Having reviewed Steps 1, 2 and 3, we are now prepared to look again at the typical day's menus, given in Table 2, and to ask ourselves whether the diet we have been following is of the order of 2500 calories, as shown in the figures on the left, or whether, through disregard of the above steps, the menu has been calorically expanded so that it approaches the figures cited on the right. To restate the above steps in succinct form: nothing is to be eaten between meals except the two glasses of milk; foods are to be selected and prepared in such a way that they will approximate the lower caloric figures cited; and finally, of course, servings are to be "average" as defined above if the values on the left are to obtain.

If these steps are followed conscientiously, the majority of expectant mothers will have no trouble with excessive weight gain even on this 2500 calorie diet. The difficulty is that many women who think they are following such a diet are actually exceeding it through "nibbles" between meals and through injudicious selection and preparation of foods.

STEP 5

But what if you belong to the small minority group in which undesirable weight gain persists despite rigorous adherence to the above suggestions? The next step is to substitute skimmed milk for the whole milk included in the above menu. This reduces forthwith the caloric content of the diet by about 300 calories — no small sum. But be sure to continue taking this quart of milk every day. It provides more protein, minerals and vitamins for less calories (and money) than any other food; and skimmed milk contains, of course, just as much protein and minerals (including calcium) as does whole milk.

STEP 6

The next step is an easy one and may well be taken simultaneously with Step 5, namely, to substitute saccharin for sugar not only in coffee or tea but for cereals and fruits. For cereals it may be dissolved in the milk used over them, and to sweeten fruits may be dissolved in a little water. Or, liquid saccharin, which can be purchased at any grocery store or food market, may be used. Saccharin should not be cooked as this makes it bitter. Step 6 will take off about 100 calories from the diet as given, possibly more. Wherever saccharin can be substituted for one level teaspoonful of sugar, twenty calories are deleted thereby — and every little bit helps.

STEP 7

Reduce drastically or eliminate altogether the salt ordinarily added to foods in the kitchen. It has been assumed all along from the suggestions made on page 70 that no salt has been employed at the table and less than usual in cooking. As already explained, there is a definite relationship between the amount of salt eaten and the amount of water retained by the body; and it is quite possible, hence, that a still further reduction in salt intake will release superfluous body water and cause a substantial weight loss. In the opinion of many physicians, rigorous limitation of salt intake not only curtails weight gain and reduces the likelihood of toxemia (see pages 117-118) but also makes for easier, quicker labors. At first this salt-poor diet may seem so bland and tasteless as to constitute something of a hardship; but it is surprising how quickly patients get used to it and after a few days, as a rule, do not object to it appreciably.

STEP 8

Eliminate the breakfast cereal and also all desserts. For the latter substitute fresh fruits sweetened, if necessary, with liquid saccharin. This should delete between 200 and 300 calories and bring the total caloric intake to something under 1900.

*   *   *   *

It is rare for expectant mothers, even though they be of rather sedentary habits, to gain excessively if they are actually, day in and day out, on a 1900 calorie diet. If, however, you have followed conscientiously the Eight Steps listed above and are still gaining more than you should, note carefully the following: *Do not attempt, on the basis of instructions or facts given in this book, or on the basis of instructions or facts given in any other book or article, to reduce your caloric intake to a level below that reached by the Eight Steps.* If these measures do not yield the desired result, you represent a special case and should be under the immediate and personal dietary supervision either of your physician or of an expert dietitian. Above all do not curtail on the Seven Basic Foods. It may possibly be that your physician or dietitian will even suggest some inroads here (particularly in the case of butter, which is the least essential of the Basic Seven), but do not take this responsibility yourself or attempt in any other way to be your own dietitian at levels under the 1900 calories cited above.

TABLE 1

Caloric Values of Nonessential Foods

Group 1 — Approximately 100 Calories

Biscuit	1 average
Carbonated drinks	6-8 ounce glass
Chocolate sauce	1 tablespoon
Cookies, most plain	1 cookie
Hollandaise sauce	1 average serving (⅛ cup)
Jell-o (plain)	½ cup scant
Junket (plain)	½ cup scant
Liquors such as rye, Scotch, gin, bourbon, brandy	1 ounce
Liqueurs	1 cordial glass
Peanut butter	1 level tablespoon
Roll	1 average
Wines (most dry)	1 wine glass

TABLE 1 (*Continued*)

Caloric Values of Nonessential Foods

Group 2 — Approximately 200 Calories

Angel food cake	About 1/12 of an average cake
Brownies	1 piece about 2″ x 2″ x 3/4″
Cake without icing	1 average slice
Cinnamon bun	1 average
Cocktails (most kinds)	1 cocktail
Cocoa	1 cup
Cornstarch puddings	1/2 cup scant
Cream puff with custard filling and thin icing	1
Cruller (no icing)	1
Doughnut (no icing)	1
Ice cream (commercial)	1/8 of a quart
Pecans, walnuts	4-6 whole nuts
Peanuts (shelled)	1 ounce
Waffle (no butter or syrup)	1 6-inch waffle
Wines (most sweet or dessert wines)	1 wine glass

TABLE 1 (*Continued*)

Caloric Values of Nonessential Foods

Group 3 — *Approximately 300 Calories*

Bread pudding with raisins	½ cup
Brown Betty	½ cup
Cream puff (no icing) with whipped cream filler	1
Cruller with icing	1
Cup cake with icing	1
Doughnut with icing	1
Fruitcake	Thin slice about ½-2 ounces
Gingerbread (no icing)	1 average serving
Ice cream (commercial)	⅙ quart
Rice pudding with raisins	½ cup

Group 4 — *Approximately 400 Calories*

Layer cake with icing	1 average slice
Pie	⅙ of a 9-inch pie
Short cakes	1 average serving

TABLE 1 (*Concluded*)

Caloric Values of Nonessential Foods

Miscellaneous

	Calories
1 piece candy (35-45 pieces per pound)	50
1 5-cent candy bar	250-400
1 piece of glacé fruit such as prune, apricot, fig	100
1 *level* tablespoon jam, jelly, marmalade, etc.	60
1 milk shake with ice cream, no whipped cream	450-500
1 level tablespoon malted milk	35-40
1 level tablespoon whipped cream	30
1 tablespoon whipping cream	75-100
Beer (1 cup)	85-150
Soups (depending on ingredients, especially amount of fat)	100-300
Most homemade cream soups per serving (⅔ cup)	200
Bouillon (canned), 1 serving	20-25
Bouillon made from 1 cube	3-6
¼ pound small link country sausage (cooked)	670
Canned fruit, 1 serving, depending upon light, medium or heavy syrup	200-300
Stewed dried fruit, 1 serving:	
Without sugar	100-200
With sugar	200-300

TABLE 2

Typical Menu

The caloric value may vary between 2500 and 3600 calories as explained in the text.

Breakfast	
	Approximate Calories
Fruit — fresh	50-100
Cereal, ¾ cup	75-100
with sugar (1 tablespoon)	60-60
and milk (½ cup)	85-85
1 egg	80-80
cooked in 1 teaspoon fat	40-40
1 slice bread	75-75
1 pat butter	60-60
Coffee: with cream (1 ounce)	60-60
with sugar (2 level teaspoons)	40-40
	625-700

Lunch	
	Approximate Calories
A main dish	200-300
Salad (vegetable, low figure; fruit, high figure)	20-100
with 1 tablespoon mayonnaise	120-120
2 slices bread	150-150
1 pat butter	60-60
Milk, 1 glass (8 ounces)	170-170
Dessert	100-200
	820-1100

TABLE 2 (*Concluded*)

4:00 P.M.

	Approximate Calories
Milk, 1 glass (8 ounces)	170-170

Dinner

	Approximate Calories
Meat, fish, poultry	200-400
Potatoes or equivalent	100-200
Green vegetable	50-100
Salad (vegetable, low figure; fruit, high figure)	20-100
with 1 tablespoon mayonnaise	120-120
Dessert	100-400
Milk, 1 glass (8 ounces)	170-170
	760-1490

Bedtime

	Approximate Calories
Milk, 1 glass (8 ounces)	170-170
Total calories for day	**2545-3630**

Chapter V

COMMON DISCOMFORTS AND
THEIR TREATMENT

Nausea. — It is common knowledge that the early weeks of pregnancy are frequently associated with some degree of nausea. In mapping out a regime to correct this tendency it is helpful to recall certain factors which predispose to nausea in the nonpregnant person, because these same factors are not uncommonly responsible for the nausea which expectant mothers experience. In the first place, as many examples show, nausea is often psychic in origin. For instance, a repellent sight, or an obnoxious odor, or the mere recollection of such a sight or odor, may give rise to nausea or even vomiting. The general use of the adjective "nauseating" to depict a repulsive object is further acknowledgment that an upset mind may produce an upset stomach. Now, in all life's encounters there are probably few experiences which are at first more upsetting, mentally and emotionally, than the realization by a young woman that she is pregnant. At the outset, there are several weeks of anxious uncertainty before she can be sure of the diagnosis. Then, no end of adjustments have to be made and plans changed. Emotionally, the implications of pregnancy extend far back into the past when she first met her husband, while its future ramifications are endless. The responsibilities entailed are plain enough also and seem on first thought, perhaps, more than can be assumed. These, and a thousand other thoughts, crowd themselves into the mind, and not infrequently the stomach, in a perverse sort of sympathy with the mind, reacts by nausea.

To ask that an expectant mother dismiss entirely from her mind the fact that she is pregnant is obviously futile, but the more she can achieve in this direction the less will she be bothered with nausea. Friends, the movies, novels, even the comic strips, are more wholesome diversions than thinking about pregnancy and should be made the most of. Above all, do not anticipate being nauseated simply because "morning sickness" is an old tradition of pregnancy. More than a third of all pregnant women escape it altogether, and with greater diversification of interests the number would doubtless be much larger.

A second circumstance which can cause nausea in the pregnant and nonpregnant alike is an empty stomach. Thus, everyone knows that the stomach is more unsettled in the morning before breakfast. This is a very important fact to bear in mind for it is the basis of the most effective treatment of the condition, namely, a regime of several small meals taken at frequent intervals so that the stomach, in so far as is possible, may never become empty. Since dry food is most easily retained, crackers and toast should be given a prominent place in the dietary program, as the following regime exemplifies:

1. Before retiring place two crackers on a table beside the bed. Upon awakening eat the crackers without rais-

ing the head from the pillows; then remain in the lying posture for twenty minutes.

2. A light breakfast, let us say brown cereal and cream, toast and coffee. Butter should not be used on the toast — marmalade, jelly or honey being substituted.

3. 10:30 A.M. Crackers or toast with a glass of milk or cup of cocoa, tea or hot malted milk.

4. Luncheon. Vegetable soup with crackers; rice, green-vegetable or fruit salad; bread or rolls.

5. 4 P.M. Crackers or toast with a glass of orange juice, grapefruit juice or lemonade.

6. Dinner. Lean meat, green vegetable, baked, boiled or mashed potatoes, rolls, tomato-and-lettuce salad, dessert.

7. Before retiring, crackers or toast with a glass of milk, or cup of cocoa, tea or hot malted milk.

It must be understood that the above dietary is only a temporary makeshift until the nausea subsides. As soon as it has definitely passed, the menu should be greatly augmented and diversified, as recommended in the previous chapter.

A third cause of nausea in both the pregnant and the nonpregnant is found in fried and greasy foods and these, together with butter, must be deleted from the diet. Likewise, cabbage, cauliflower and spinach are often upsetting. Although water may prove to be troublesome, every effort should be made to consume the equivalent of six glasses of fluid a day in some form, such as cocoa, milk, soups, or ginger ale. Since substances in the wheat germ are believed to exert a particularly salutary effect on nausea in pregnancy, whole-bread and cereals should be incorporated in each day's menu.

Relief from nausea is often obtained by lying down and it is a good plan to do this whenever the sensation comes on. Some women, indeed, find that the discomfort can be forestalled altogether by lying down regularly for twenty minutes immediately after each meal. The beneficial effect of the horizontal posture is often enhanced by placing an ice bag over the region of the stomach, or a towel wrung out in cold water.

In the vast majority of cases the measures outlined above, if followed meticulously, will put an end to the nausea. If they do not — particularly if the condition is associated with actual vomiting — the condition should be reported to your medical attendant.

Heartburn. — By heartburn is meant a burning sensation in the upper abdomen or lower part of the chest, sometimes associated with the belching of small amounts of bitter fluid. It has nothing to do with the heart, but results from sluggish intestinal activity and is actually a mild form of indigestion. In view of this fact, the first step in the treatment of the condition should be a careful survey of one's dietary habits to make sure that rich and indigestible foods are omitted and that overeating and hurried eating are avoided. Oddly enough, the best preventive measure entails the use of a rich food, but one taken at a specific time, that is, one tablespoonful of cream thirty minutes before meals. Once the heartburn has started, this procedure is of no value whatsoever; taken along with meals, moreover, this amount of fat would tend to aggravate rather than to relieve heartburn, but when taken a short while before meals a tablespoonful of cream tends to stimulate intestinal activity, and so eliminates the cause of the discomfort. Relief from heartburn is most readily obtained by taking a level teaspoonful of milk of magnesia. Some women seem to be relieved by chewing gum. *Do not* take baking soda (sodium bicarbonate).

Flatulence. — Distention of the stomach and intestines with gas, a condition known to doctors as "flatulence," may accompany heartburn or appear independently. It is usually due to undesirable bacterial action in the intestines superimposed on the circumstance that the pressure of the enlarged uterus hinders the intestinal contents from moving along as rapidly as usual. Because of the latter fact, the primary consideration in the treatment of flatulence is regular evacuation of the bowels. Another important preventive measure is to chew all solid food very slowly and thoroughly. At the same time care should be taken to avoid gas-producing foods such as beans, parsnips, corn, onions, cabbage, fried foods and sweet desserts. Some women find it helpful to have their vegetables puréed.

Constipation. — Many women who have always been quite regular become constipated in pregnancy because of the pressure of the enlarged uterus on the lower intestine. Since it is necessary for the expectant mother to eliminate the waste products of the fetus as well as her own, a daily bowel movement is essential. This may often be expedited by a few simple measures such as the following:

1. Upon arising drink a glass or two of cold water.

While hot water may be substituted if desired, cold has a more stimulating effect on the digestive tract. A few drops of lemon juice may make the drink more refreshing.

2. Eat a coarse cereal such as oatmeal for breakfast. Do not, however, go to the extreme of eating bran breakfast foods, which are irritating to the stomach and intestine and often cause indigestion. Marmalade with breakfast is beneficial, since its juices are laxative and the pieces of hard orange skin act as a mechanical stimulus to the bowel.

3. Eat some fruit at night before going to bed. Fruits are helpful not only in adding bulk to the stool, but because their juices contain various acids, sugars and salts which are laxative. Certain fruits, of course, are particularly efficacious, notably prunes, figs, raisins, dates and apples. Prunes enjoy a well-deserved reputation as laxative agents and a small quantity of prune juice at night may be all that is necessary.

4. Eat plentifully of green vegetables, both raw and cooked. These add so-called roughage to the stool and thereby stimulate the eliminative action of the intestines. Whole-wheat bread has the same tendency and should be used instead of white bread.

5. Make a habit of going to the toilet at a regular time, preferably after breakfast.

6. Most physicians have no objection to the expectant mother's taking milk of magnesia, a tablespoonful at bedtime, but she should employ no other laxative without her doctor's advice.

Hemorrhoids (Piles). — These are collections of large veins at the opening of the rectum. Pregnancy predisposes to their development because the growing uterus tends to obstruct the blood flow in the region of the rectum and thus interferes with the emptying of the veins. Pregnancy alone, however, does not actually produce hemorrhoids unless constipation is present, because the two essential causes are hard stools and straining at stool. Under these circumstances the veins become enlarged, stretched and painful; not infrequently the condition is associated with itching and slight bleeding. It is only common sense, therefore, that the first step in the treatment of the hemorrhoids is correction of constipation.

Pending advice from your physician, painful hemorrhoids are best treated as follows: Lie down with the hips slightly elevated and apply to the rectal region a cloth or strip of gauze which has been soaked either in ice water or in iced witch hazel. These dressings should be changed frequently in order that they may be kept constantly wet and cold. Sometimes hot applications afford more relief than cold. Ointments, with the exception of cold cream which is often soothing, should be used only on the doctor's advice.

Varicose Veins. — Just as the enlarged uterus tends to obstruct blood flow from the rectal region and thereby predisposes to hemorrhoids, so it may likewise interfere with blood flow from the lower extremities and give rise to swollen veins in the legs. Varicose veins are not likely to develop in the course of a first pregnancy, but may be very annoying in women who have had previous children. As we have said, circular garters and rolled stockings aggravate any tendency in this direction and must not be used. The treatment is of two kinds. In the first place, every opportunity should be seized to elevate the leg on a pillow so that the heel is slightly higher than the hip; the more this is done at odd times in the day and evening, the better. Second, if this simple postural treatment is insufficient, an elastic bandage or stocking must be worn. Elastic bandages may be purchased at most drugstores, are just as effective as stockings and are decidedly cheaper. The stockings possess the advantage that they are easier to put on, are neater and will not become disarranged and slip down as the bandages are likely to do. Whether bandages or stockings are used, they must be applied in the morning before arising. In this way support is given to the veins at a time when they are well emptied from the night's elevation of the leg; these measures are of no value when employed after the veins have had an opportunity to fill.

It must be understood that "elastic bandages" are especially made for the relief of varicose veins and that ordinary bandage material is of no value for this purpose. The most satisfactory bandages are made of elastic webbing rather than rubber; they are usually about three inches wide and some three yards long. In applying the bandage one or two turns should first be wound around the foot; it is then wound spirally around the ankle and thence up the leg, with firm pressure, to a point slightly above the highest varicose vein; the turns should overlap by about one inch and the upper end be secured with a safety pin. The bandage should be worn all day and removed at night. Upon being washed, it regains its original elasticity.

Muscular Cramps. — During the later weeks of pregnancy, muscular cramps in the back and thighs are a common cause of discomfort. As we have seen, the enlarged, protruding uterus calls for a backward tilt of the torso if equilibrium is to be maintained — a posture which imposes a constant strain on the back and thigh muscles whenever the woman is on her feet. It follows, therefore, that adequate amounts of rest are the best preventive. A well-fitting maternity corset and moderately low heels, as previously emphasized, are also beneficial. A considerable degree of immediate relief may be obtained by massage of the group of muscles involved, using olive oil or cold cream as a lubricant. In this connection it is interesting to recall that liniments by the carload have been sold by patent medicine companies with the claim that they are specific for this very trouble. They are of no value, since it is the massage employed in rubbing the liniment in which is efficacious, not any magic drug in the liniment. Shooting pains down the legs are not infrequently due to pressure of the baby's head on certain nerves and are often relieved by a change in position; if pains of this type are severe, it may even be worthwhile to try the knee-chest position for a few minutes (page 190).

Fainting. — Dizzy spells and actual fainting attacks are experienced by a few women, particularly during the first half of pregnancy. They are not serious and usually ameliorate as time goes on, but they should be reported to your physician. If you are subject to these, it is advisable to carry with you a small bottle of aromatic spirits of ammonia or of smelling salts; a quick whiff of either of these will usually ward off an attack.

Shortness of Breath. — As a result of the upward pressure of the enlarged uterus against the lungs, shortness of breath is common during the last two months. In first pregnancies, decided relief is usually experienced a week or two before confinement because the baby's head sinks into the pelvis, thereby giving more room above. If shortness of breath interferes with sleep, the head and shoulders should be comfortably propped up with several pillows so that a semi-sitting posture is assumed. Almost invariably this relieves shortness of breath to the extent that a restful night's sleep may be had. Although some shortness of breath is perfectly normal in the later weeks of pregnancy, it should be reported to your physician if it reaches such a degree that you cannot climb a flight of stairs without discomfort.

Insomnia. — Although the early part of pregnancy is often accompanied by an overpowering desire to sleep, the later weeks are sometimes associated with insomnia. Many factors contribute to this, including movements of the baby, shortness of breath and muscular cramps — to say nothing of thoughts about the coming infant. A short walk in the open air before bedtime, followed by a warm sponge bath or shower and a cup of hot cocoa or milk, will often meet the difficulty. You may sleep in any position in which you are comfortable for there is no possibility of "compressing" the baby; a hot-water bottle to the feet or an extra pillow under the head may help. Not a few women require a mild sedative now and then in the last few weeks of pregnancy, but this should be taken only on the advice of your physician.

Vaginal Discharge. — Moderate vaginal discharge, even enough to necessitate wearing a pad, is common in the later part of pregnancy because of seepage of fluids from the congested and succulent vagina and neck of the uterus. It is ordinarily pale yellow in color and thin. If thick in consistency or very profuse, or if associated with itching, it should be reported to the physician who will institute suitable treatment. In most cases external cleansing of the parts with warm water is all that is necessary. As we have already emphasized, douches must not be taken unless detailed instructions are received from your doctor.

Chapter VI

DANGER SIGNALS

IF you have ever grown flowers, you will recall that even in the best-kept garden an occasional sprout will show signs of blight, evidence that something is interfering with the normal process of plant reproduction. You will also realize that if this plant is properly sprayed, at the very first signs of the fungus infection, the disease is eradicated and the sprout develops normally; whereas if the blight is allowed to progress untreated, havoc may result. Now let us suppose that we had an expert horticulturist in charge of our hypothetical garden, one who would diligently and at frequent intervals inspect each sprout, and, at the very first sign of trouble, institute with professional skill the type of treatment which his long experience told him was best. Surely, then, there would be no cause to worry about our flowers! In human reproduction the situation is similar, for here also things sometimes go amiss, but here, likewise, early recognition by a trained observer together with intelligent treatment usually results in cure. Very often the expectant mother is not aware of these disturbances and in the early stages of certain common complications may feel quite well. Only the physician's careful examination can detect the beginning of these disturbances and only by making her visits to his office with punctilious regularity can she be certain that deviations from the normal will be detected at their onset and as quickly corrected.

Sometimes, between visits to her doctor, the expectant mother may notice certain changes in her condition which merit reporting to the physician at once. More often than not, these findings observed by the patient prove to be of no significance; nevertheless, the physician should be notified without delay in order that he may inquire into their circumstances, decide whether they are real danger signals or not, and, if they seem to be, institute treatment. THE FOLLOWING SYMPTOMS DEMAND IMMEDIATE REPORT TO THE DOCTOR:

1. VAGINAL BLEEDING, NO MATTER HOW SLIGHT.
2. SWELLING OF THE FACE OR FINGERS.
3. SEVERE, CONTINUOUS HEADACHE.
4. DIMNESS OR BLURRING OF VISION.
5. PAIN IN THE ABDOMEN.
6. PERSISTENT VOMITING.
7. CHILLS AND FEVER.
8. SUDDEN ESCAPE OF WATER FROM THE VAGINA.

Although these symptoms may sound formidable, their significance depends entirely on the circumstances under which they occur. Even the development of several of them may be quite in keeping with the normal state of affairs and is not necessarily a cause for concern. For instance, the onset of normal labor is often heralded by a very slight amount of bleeding, recurrent pain in the abdomen and a discharge of water from the vagina. In the main, however, these symptoms deserve particular

attention because they often constitute warning signs of
the three most common complications of pregnancy,
namely: miscarriage, toxemia and pyelitis. It is true that
there are other complications of pregnancy, but they are
so rare that the chance of the average woman experiencing any one of them is less than one in two hundred. In
view of this fact, let us limit our discussion to these
three more common conditions.

Miscarriage. — The word "miscarriage" as used by the
laity means the birth of the fetus before it is sufficiently
developed to live outside of the mother's body, that is,
before the seventh lunar month of pregnancy. Doctors,
however, rarely employ this term, but refer to the accident ordinarily as an "abortion." It must be understood
that the word "abortion," as used in medical terminology,
carries no implication whatsoever that the condition
was produced intentionally; in other words, the doctors'
term "abortion" and the laity's word "miscarriage" are
practically synonymous. Accordingly, if your doctor inquires if you have ever had an abortion, be not dismayed
or offended; he is simply asking if you have ever had a
miscarriage, that is, a previous pregnancy which termi-
nated of its own accord in the early months. When physicians wish to indicate that the event was brought on intentionally, they speak either of a "criminal abortion"
(meaning that it was effected illegally without justifiable
reason), or of a "therapeutic abortion" (meaning that it
was produced ethically because of some grave maternal
disease which made continuation of the pregnancy extremely hazardous).

Miscarriages are very common, reliable estimates showing that at least one pregnancy in every ten terminates, of its own accord, in this manner. Most miscarriages occur during the second and third months; thereafter the likelihood of the accident is decidedly less. What causes all these miscarriages — so tragic and shattering to so many women? Is Mother Nature actually as cruel to our mothers as these figures would suggest? If we review the situation with some perspective and with full fairness to all concerned, we must arrive at the inevitable conclusion that most of these miscarriages, far from being tragedies, are blessings in disguise, for they are Nature's beneficent way of extinguishing an embryo which is imperfect. This is particularly true of very early miscarriages. Indeed, careful microscopic study of the material passed shows that in 80 per cent of these some defect is present in the embryo which is either incompatible with life or would result in a grossly deformed child. The incidence of abnormalities in embryos passed after the second month is somewhat lower, but not less than 50 per cent. Some authorities believe that 80 per cent of all miscarriages are ascribable to this cause. Whether the female or male germ cell is at fault in these cases it is usually difficult, if not impossible, to say; either may be responsible. Miscarriages of this sort are obviously unpreventable and, although bitterly disappointing to the parents, serve in the long run a useful purpose.

Since imperfectly formed embryos are almost always aborted early in pregnancy, the likelihood of a full-term child's being defective is very remote. Not a few expectant mothers worry about this possibility as the time of

confinement approaches, but such fears are quite unjusti-
fied. If the child is carried beyond the second half of
pregnancy, the chances are fifty to one that he will be
born without the slightest blemish.

Although many miscarriages are due to factors other
than defects in the embryo, little is known about these
causes. In certain cases the uterus happens to be tilted
backward and this condition may occasionally cause the
accident. If this be true, an early visit to the physician
will result in detection and correction of the malposition
and consequently a better outlook. Many women are
wont to explain miscarriage on the grounds of injury of
one type or another, or excessive activity. Different
women exhibit the greatest variation in this respect. In
some, the pregnancy may go blithely on despite falls
from second-story windows and automobile accidents so
severe as to fracture the hip bone. In others, a trivial
fall or just overfatigue seems to produce miscarriage.
Since there is no way of foretelling who is susceptible to
the accident and who is not, it would seem prudent for
every expectant mother to follow the dictates of common
sense and avoid long automobile trips, lifting heavy
weights and any form of activity which involves jolting.

The first symptom of impending miscarriage is usually
bleeding. In some cases this begins as a little irregular
spotting, followed in a day or two by a moderate discharge of blood which simulates a menstrual period;
this state of affairs may persist for several weeks before
the onset of pain and increased bleeding denotes the
beginning of the process by which the product of conception is expelled. In other cases the bleeding may be

profuse from the start and accompanied by recurrent cramplike pains, similar to those experienced sometimes during menstruation. Occasionally, pain is the first symptom of miscarriage, but in most cases, it is preceded by bleeding.

At the first sign of bleeding — even the slightest spotting — the patient should go to bed at once and have her doctor notified. His observations may reveal the fact that the condition is simply a threatened miscarriage. In that case, rest in bed and certain medication may halt the process; with suitable rest and care, many women have gone through pregnancy quite successfully after such an experience. In some instances, however, the bleeding defies all efforts to stop it, the pain augments and the product of conception is expelled. If it is passed completely, a suitable period of rest in bed, as specified by the doctor, terminates the episode. It frequently happens, however, that only part of the product of conception is passed. In that event, depending on the amount of bleeding and other factors, it sometimes becomes necessary for the doctor to remove the remainder. This procedure requires but a few minutes, is not a serious operation and, being done under anesthesia, is altogether painless. Since the treatment of any case of miscarriage depends in large measure on the completeness with which the product of conception has been expelled, it is extremely important that all material passed, including blood clots, be saved for the doctor to examine.

Miscarriages which start of their own accord and receive proper treatment are rarely serious in so far as the mother's physical welfare is concerned. To be sure, rumors to the contrary are occasionally heard, but if these are traced down, it will usually be found that they refer to the dire results which ensue when the woman herself, or some illicit practitioner or midwife, provokes the process intentionally. Unless the mother's health is at stake, no reputable member of the profession would undertake such a procedure, for it constitutes murder; consequently, these clandestine operations are usually performed by hands which are not only unskilled but unclean. The results, all too often, are unbelievably tragic. Accustomed though we may be in this age of machinery, science and "free thought" to disregard natural phenomena, pregnancy is one process of nature with which it is best not to tamper.

Every year huge quantities of castor oil, quinine and other "powerful" drugs are sold for the express purpose of interrupting early pregnancy. As a rule, these concoctions merely produce nausea and vomiting, while pregnancy goes nonchalantly on; certain of the patent medicines sold for this purpose, however, contain ingredients which act with such violence that hemorrhages into the bowel and kidneys sometimes ensue with results that may be exceedingly grave. The reputation of these drugs rests on the circumstance that the menstrual interval in the same woman often varies widely; as we have said, a woman who has been accustomed to menstruate every twenty-eight days may occasionally experience a thirty-five-day cycle without apparent cause or detriment to health. If, in such a long cycle, when she thinks herself five or six days "overdue," she takes one of these medicines and starts menstruating the next day, the drug is naturally acclaimed as the benefactor. It is obvious that the same end would have been attained had she done nothing. At the present writing, there is no drug known to the medical profession which will produce miscarriage in the human being, whether given by mouth or by injection.

Toxemia. — During the latter part of pregnancy, for reasons that are unknown, the expectant mother occasionally manifests a group of signs and symptoms which are called by physicians "toxemia." Although by derivation the word means "poison in the blood," no such poison has been demonstrated and it is generally agreed that this appellation is a misnomer. In the majority of cases, the patient at first feels quite well but shows, on medical examination, an increase in the blood pressure; along with this, albumin may appear in the urine, a finding indicative of a kidney disturbance. The chief symptoms which the mother, herself, may notice include: swelling of the face and fingers (are the eyes swollen in the morning? is the wedding ring tight?), rapid gain in weight (bathroom scales are an asset throughout pregnancy), persistent headache not amenable to the usual methods of treatment and difficulty with the eyes such as blurring of vision. If the condition is properly treated, no harm comes to either mother or child, all these signs and symptoms disappearing entirely, as a rule, after the baby is born, but if it is neglected, serious complications may ensue. It is important that the expectant mother should be cognizant of the toxemias of pregnancy for a number of reasons. She will understand, in the first place, why frequent blood pressure determinations are desirable during

the later months. Second, in the event that a slight elevation of blood pressure should occur, she will appreciate
the necessity of exact compliance with the doctor's instructions and will not minimize their importance merely
because she "feels well"; paradoxically enough, a woman
may "feel well" and yet be decidedly ill from toxemia.
And finally, of course, she will realize the importance of
communicating at once with her physician in case any of
the symptoms mentioned above develop.

The treatment of toxemia of pregnancy depends so
much upon the circumstances of each individual case
that it is possible here to mention only two phases of it,
namely, diminution of salt intake and rest. Concerning
the desirability of the former measure, physicians are in
general agreement, particularly if there is a tendency for
the hands and face to swell. Some physicians recommend
that no additional salt be added at the table, many others that no salt whatsoever be used in cooking. Although
the latter omission makes foods somewhat tasteless at
first, the palate becomes adjusted to the change in a
surprisingly short time so that food prepared in this way
becomes just as inviting as artificially salted food. As mentioned previously, the salt naturally present in most foodstuffs is ample for body requirements. Another important
form of treatment in toxemia is rest. Not infrequently
complete rest in bed is desirable; and to this end, physicians often suggest a few days' stay in the hospital not
only for the purpose of absolute rest but also in order
that meticulous surveillance may be exercised over diet,
fluid intake, weight control and other essentials of treatment.

Pyelitis. — The kidney pelvis, the funnel-like portion of the kidney which conveys the urine from the kidney to the tube (the ureter) leading to the bladder, is a common site of inflammation in pregnancy. This condition, known as pyelitis, occurs about once in every fifty pregnancies; it is most likely to develop about the sixth month, but may make its appearance at any time in pregnancy. When it is recalled that the enlarged uterus presses backward against the ureter, it is easy to understand that the flow of urine through it could readily be impeded and that a certain degree of damming back of urine might result. When the flow of urine through the kidney pelvis and ureter is not brisk, stagnation is prone to ensue with consequent inflammation. The characteristic symptoms of pyelitis are chills, fever and pain in one or another flank, most frequently the right. Pyelitis is rarely a serious condition and, as a rule, responds readily to treatment. The most important thing for the expectant mother to know about pyelitis is that copious water drinking, six or eight glasses a day, by continually flushing out the kidneys is a valuable preventive and renders the development of the condition most unlikely.

THE Rh FACTOR

The Rh factor is a certain substance which most people have in their blood. It derives its name from the first two letters of the scientific term for the common monkey, the rhesus monkey, in the blood of which the factor is always present. The exact proportion of the white race which have the Rh factor is about 85 per cent; these people are called Rh positive. The remaining 15 per cent, who are without the factor, are called Rh negative.[1]

When the blood of an Rh positive person is introduced, through blood transfusion or otherwise, into the blood stream of an Rh negative individual, the latter develops antibodies against the Rh factor present in the blood administered. Antibodies are substances which the body manufactures as a protective mechanism to counteract the effect of various kinds of new materials which may be introduced into the blood and tissues. For instance, when bacteria gain access to the blood stream, antibodies against that particular kind of bacteria are usually developed and, sooner or later, destroy the bacteria. Antibodies may be regarded, accordingly, as a sort of defensive army which the blood and tissues muster against foreign, invading forces. It is these antibodies which cure most bacterial diseases from the common cold to typhoid fever. Moreover, they often remain present in the blood and tissues long after the disease has been successfully combated, making the person immune to that particular type of infection; in other words, should the same bacterium or material which incited the original manufacture of the antibodies be again introduced into the body, these defensive substances now stand ready to attack and destroy it.

As stated above, when an Rh negative person is given a blood transfusion from an Rh positive donor, antibodies are developed by the recipient against the Rh substance present in the administered blood. But, as is

[1] Only 7 per cent of Negroes are Rh negative, about 1 per cent of Chinese.

true when bacteria invade the body, these antibodies against the Rh factor do not form instantaneously, but only after a period of time. Consequently, with the first transfusion, nothing out of the ordinary occurs. However, should this Rh negative recipient receive at some later date another transfusion from an Rh positive donor, antibodies will probably have been developed and these will immediately attack the Rh factor. Since the Rh substance is an integral part of the red blood cells, this "battle" causes a violent commotion in the blood stream with the destruction of many red cells. As the broken-down products of these fragmented red cells are disseminated throughout the body, they exert a poisonous effect and as a result the recipient of the blood transfusion suffers a reaction usually manifested by a chill and fever but sometimes by more grave symptoms. In World War II, when many Rh negative soldiers had to be given repeated blood transfusions, this Rh problem was a serious one. It was met by using Rh negative donors for transfusions of Rh negative persons — in other words, by administering blood without any Rh factor in it to cause the trouble described above. Nowadays physicians and surgeons everywhere are careful to determine the Rh status of any prospective recipient of a blood transfusion; if it is negative, blood from an Rh negative donor is employed.

But what has all this to do with pregnancy? Once in every several hundred pregnancies, as the result of an extraordinary combination of chance factors, the Rh substance may be responsible for a chain of events which exerts a harmful effect on the fetus. A number of circumstances must be present before this singular action on the fetus can be exerted, as follows: In the first place, the woman must be Rh negative; as indicated above, there is only one chance in seven that any member of the white race belongs to this minority group. In the second place, her husband must be Rh positive; the chances are good — six out of seven — that he does belong to the positive group, but he may not. In the third place, the fetus must be Rh positive; just because the husband is Rh positive it does not necessarily follow that the baby is positive, because if any large group of Rh positive men are studied it will be found that the spermatozoa of about one fourth are Rh negative and will produce an Rh negative infant. In the fourth place — and this is the most unlikely circumstance in the lot — the Rh substance from the Rh positive fetus must find its way through the placenta and into the blood stream of the mother and build up antibodies therein just as occurs with an Rh positive blood transfusion. Once these antibodies are developed in the mother they pass through the placenta into the fetal blood stream where they cause varying degrees of damage to the infant's red blood cells. Finally, the woman must have had a previous pregnancy or a previous blood transfusion because, as we have seen, it takes some time for the antibodies to develop.

From the above facts the following rather comforting conclusions can be drawn. Six out of seven women are Rh positive and for them there is no possibility whatsoever of complications occurring from this source. Likewise in first pregnancies, even if the expectant mother is Rh negative, the possibility of trouble developing is practically nil unless she has had a previous blood transfusion with Rh positive blood. But if a woman is Rh negative and has had previous pregnancies or previous transfusions, what is her outlook in subsequent pregnancies? So many factors enter into this question that it is impossible to answer it with great precision, but all authorities agree that the vast majority even of this group — 90 to 95 per cent — go through pregnancy after pregnancy without any suggestion of a complication.

But if all this be true, why has so much space been devoted to the Rh factor in this book? Simply to set the truth against the many grossly exaggerated, grossly distorted and often grossly inaccurate tales about the Rh factor which have appeared in some of our leading lay magazines. The authors of these reports, in order to give their articles "popular appeal," have chosen to concentrate on the dramatic, the morbid and lurid; and understatements are not their wont. They usually neglect, moreover, to mention how infrequently this trouble arises. Moreover, even if it does arise, prompt pediatric care and blood transfusion save 95 per cent of the affected, live-born infants. Let it be emphasized that the mathematical chances of the expectant mother who is reading these lines losing a baby from Rh complications — and this statement is based on the most modern, authoritative figures — is of the order of 1 in 500.

HOW TO TELEPHONE YOUR DOCTOR

If it becomes desirable to telephone your physician in order to report one or another symptom or make inquiries about it, bear in mind the following suggestions:

1. If the reason for the telephone call is vaginal bleeding in pregnancy or a discharge of water from the vagina, it is advisable to go to bed, pending word from the physician, and have your husband or someone else telephone. But be sure to have the person making the call well informed about details. For instance, if the condition prompting the call is vaginal bleeding in pregnancy, how much blood is being passed? Is it mere spotting mixed with mucus? Is it as much as occurs on the first day of a menstrual period, or more, or less? Has there been any pain associated with the bleeding? If so, is it in the midline and cramplike in character or is it to one or another side of the abdomen? If you are so fortunate as to have a telephone at your bedside, make the call yourself.

2. Under all other circumstances, talk to the doctor yourself if at all possible. To relay questions and answers back and forth through a third party is not only likely to result in a misleading story for the doctor, and garbled advice for you, but trebles the time consumed by the call.

3. Provided the condition prompting the call is not one of the danger signals listed on page 111, call the physician's office during usual office hours.

4. Do not ask offhand to speak to the doctor but report the reason for your call to the secretary or nurse who answers the phone. If the matter you have in mind is a very routine one, the secretary or nurse can often answer it to your complete satisfaction; or she may be able to ask the physician about it at a more convenient moment and call you back. If the reason for your call is not so

simple that it can be handled in one of the above ways, rest assured that the doctor will either speak to you at once or call you back very shortly.

5. Have paper and pencil at hand when you make the call. Do not waste precious moments looking for these articles after you have the physician on the phone.

6. If you are calling about any symptom that has developed, know the name, address and telephone number of your nearest pharmacy. Not infrequently the physician will want to telephone a prescription for you to that pharmacy; and obviously it will expedite matters if you can give the phone number.

Chapter VII

PREPARATIONS FOR
THE BABY

THE preparation of the baby's layette is naturally an important and enjoyable undertaking for every expectant mother. Fortunately for all concerned, the dictates of common sense have greatly simplified this problem in recent years and today chief emphasis is laid on certain practical considerations, namely, that the clothes should be comfortable for the baby and time-saving for the mother. They must be loose, of course, permitting complete freedom of motion. They should be light in weight and not too warm; particularly in steam-heated apartments, the common tendency is to dress the baby too heavily, an error which often gives rise to skin irritation as well as to fretfulness. From everyone's point of view, including that of the father, the clothes should be easy to put on and take off; the time has passed when the father can side-step the chore of changing the baby's clothes simply because he does not know how; the baby, too, will appreciate such arrangements because prolonged handling is tiring.

In the main, the tendency is to buy too much rather than too little. The following three lists comprise all that is necessary to have ready, but they may be supplemented or modified, according to individual taste.

THE LAYETTE

4 or 5 Undershirts. Cotton knit, 6 months size.

4 to 6 Kimonos. These are nowadays preferred to dresses.

4 Cotton Knit Nightgowns. These usually have a drawstring in the sleeves and at the bottom so that the baby's hands and feet will not be chilled if he becomes uncovered during the night.

2 Blanket-weight Sleeping Bags. These take the place of blankets and are much more efficacious in keeping the baby warm on cold nights.

2 Pairs Bootees. For occasional use.

2 Pairs Socks. For occasional use.

2 Sacques or Sweaters. These should open down the front.

1 Cap and Coat or Bunting.

3 Dozen Diapers. A few years ago no description of diapers would have been necessary as there was only one kind, made of bird's-eye, 22 x 22 inches. Today there are several ways of meeting this problem. The old-fashioned bird's-eye diaper is still satisfactory and the most widely used. Among new varieties there is one very popular type made of a fine, porous webbing which is folded, according to lines woven in the material, in such a way that it is put on like a pair of drawers and protection is given where most needed. There are also several kinds of sanitary diapers which are made to be thrown away after using. These are especially good for travel. Then, too, in most large cities there are diaper laundering services, similar to towel laundering services, which are extremely convenient. Nothing is bought; but for a certain fee, clean, sterilized diapers are delivered daily and the soiled ones collected. When available, this service relieves the mother of much tiresome and messy work. But, even if you employ diaper service, it is prudent to have a dozen of your own on hand, "just in case."

2 Pairs Waterproof Pants. These can be of rubber, silk or plastic.

4 to 6 Bibs. For feedings and teething.

2 Dresses. These are unnecessary but may be useful for special occasions and for the sake of a change. Attractive dresses of nainsook or dimity, within a large price range, may be obtained at all department stores; or, if preferred, patterns may be purchased and the garments made.

2 Petticoats. For use with dresses. Nainsook is the material most commonly employed.

NURSERY NEEDS

1 Bed or Basket.

1 Mattress.

6 Sheets. Cotton knit sheets are convenient since ironing is not necessary. Fitted crib sheets, with corners made to fit over and under the four corners of the mattress, are readily available, simplify bed making and provide a wrinkle-proof surface.

2 Large Rubber Sheets. These are to be placed between the mattress and the sheet and should be of sufficient size to be tucked under the mattress.

6 Crib Pads. These are to be put under the baby, should be quilted or made of Turkish toweling and should measure about 18 x 18 inches.

1 Woolen Crib Blanket. This must be large enough to tuck under the baby's mattress.

4-6 Receiving Blankets.

1 Dressing Table or Bathinette. This is invaluable for bathing, dressing and changing the baby. Several folding types with plastic top, plastic bathtub and pockets for accessories are available at department stores.

1 Pair Scales. Balance or beam scales, equipped with a basket, are preferable. With spring scales the dial hand vibrates whenever the baby wriggles and accurate weighing is almost impossible.

BABY'S TRAY

3 Nursing Bottles (8-ounce, Pyrex). More will be required if baby is bottle-fed. The new pre-sterilized, disposable "inner bottles" possess certain advantages but are somewhat expensive.

6 Nipples.

1 Nipple Jar.

1 Bottle Brush.

3 Covered Jars. For cotton balls and cotton swabs.

Safety Pins (large and small). A bar of soap makes an excellent "safety-pin cushion" for, by lubricating the points of the pins, it facilitates inserting them into the diapers.

Absorbent Cotton.

Soap.
Baby Oil and Talcum.
4 Wash Cloths (knitted, smooth).
2 Hand Towels (knitted, smooth).
2 Bath Towels (knitted, smooth).

Chapter VIII

THE BIRTH OF THE BABY

Hospital Delivery. — More than 95 per cent of the births in the United States now take place in hospitals; hence, the problem of hospital versus home delivery is no longer much of a question. Nevertheless, since occasional expectant mothers have the notion that home delivery might be advantageous and since several magazine articles have advanced the same thought, it would seem appropriate to review the whys and wherefores of hospital delivery.

The modern trend toward hospitalization for childbirth, a trend that has gained ground every year, is a development of the past three decades. In the early years of this century it was well-nigh impossible to persuade a respectable woman to enter a hospital for normal delivery, since only the derelicts of womankind and the destitute sought hospitalization for such a purpose. The present popularity of the hospital, then, has been achieved against great odds and can only mean that hospital care has proved its value to millions of satisfied mothers. It is often said that doctors are largely responsible for this change because of the great convenience which accrues to them. While this has doubtless been an important factor, the change could not have been brought about unless the mothers themselves had been in hearty accord. Women who have had one baby at home and another in the hospital almost always affirm that hospital delivery is more comfortable, more restful and, as a rule, only slightly more expensive. The bother and expense of preparing the rather complicated paraphernalia necessary for home confinement are avoided; the salary and board of a nurse are spared and, as well, a considerable outlay for laundry; furthermore, a period of complete rest is assured without a responsibility in the world. But most important of all is the safety offered by hospitals in the event any slight complication develops. Their laboratory facilities, their special apparatus, to say nothing of their greatest pillar of security, the staff of nurses and doctors, make modern hospitals the very safest place in the world to have a baby.

Things to Take to the Hospital. — With few exceptions, hospitals provide everything needed for the baby during his stay in the hospital. A home-going outfit will be required, of course, but whether this is taken to the hospital along with your own things or brought later by your husband is a matter of personal convenience. Nor will you, yourself, need very much; but it is a matter of experience that a hospital stay is somewhat more comfortable if you pack in your bag, preferably a month or so before the expected day of confinement, the following articles:

Comb, brush and hand-mirror.
Toothbrush and paste.
Talcum powder. For yourself — your favorite kind.
Cologne or toilet water.

Cosmetics.

Manicure set.

Sanitary belt. Pads are furnished by hospital.

Gowns. Hospital gowns are preferable the first few days
and may be worn throughout if desired, but after a
day or two most women prefer their own, which, to
say the least, are more attractive than those furnished
by the hospital. Many women prefer pajama tops to
gowns; they are certainly more practical during the
stay in bed.

Bed jacket.	*Fountain pen, stationery*
Dressing robe.	*and stamps.*
Bedroom slippers.	*A book or two.*
Clock or watch.	*Handkerchiefs or tissues.*

*Also, clothes for baby on trip home, according to time of
year.*

Lightening. — During the last few weeks of pregnancy
a number of changes indicate that the coming of the infant is not far off. In a woman having her first baby, the
uterus sinks downward and forward, an alteration which
relieves abdominal pressure, makes breathing easier and
consequently has been called "lightening." This may
occur at any time during the last four weeks, but occasionally does not eventuate until labor has actually begun. This sinking of the uterus is the result of the passage of the baby's head into the pelvic cavity and, in a
sense, is the first step in the expulsion of the child. Lightening often occurs suddenly, so that the expectant
mother arises one morning entirely relieved of the abdominal tightness and pressure which she has previ-

ously experienced. But the relief in one direction is often followed by signs of greater pressure below, particularly shooting pains down the legs and an increase in the amount of vaginal discharge. In women who have had previous children lightening occasionally takes place during the last week or ten days of pregnancy, but is more likely to occur after labor begins.

How to Tell When Labor Begins. — The onset of labor is heralded by one or more of three signs:

1. Painful, recurrent contractions of the uterus (labor pains).
2. Passage of a small amount of blood-tinged mucus ("show").
3. Passage, usually a gush, of water from the vagina (rupture of the bag of waters, or membranes).

Contractions of the uterus occur from time to time throughout pregnancy as evidenced by the fact that the organ now and then assumes a woody hardness. These contractions, however, are painless and most irregular in the time of their occurrence. True labor pains are quite different from these and may usually be identified by several characteristics. In the first place, they are painful. At the onset of labor the pain is usually located in the small of the back, but after a few hours it tends to radiate girdlewise to the front. As a rule the pain begins as a slight twinge of backache, augments in crescendo fashion, reaches an acme which is maintained a few seconds and then diminishes gradually; in the opinion of many women it is not unlike a severe menstrual cramp. The duration of such a pain, as well as its intensity, varies according to the stage of labor; at the outset it may not last longer than thirty seconds; later its length may range between a minute and a minute and a half. A particularly important characteristic of true labor pains is their rhythmicity. Even at the beginning of labor they are spaced at fairly regular intervals of fifteen to twenty minutes, the intervening periods being entirely free from pain. As labor progresses the pains become closer together and within a few hours the interval is usually in the neighborhood of five minutes. Since any muscle becomes hard when it contracts, labor pains are always associated with a hardness of the uterus. This change may be readily felt by placing the hand on the abdomen during a pain.

In some instances the expectant mother complains of pains which seem to fill all the criteria of true labor pains but which, instead of becoming harder and more frequent, diminish in intensity after a few hours and finally disappear altogether. These "false pains" are a nuisance to patient and physician alike since they are often difficult to distinguish from true labor. Indeed, maternity hospitals the country over are continually admitting patients who seem to everyone concerned to be in real labor but who report, after a short while, that their pains have entirely stopped; the patient then returns home to find that days or even weeks may elapse before effectual labor sets in; on the other hand, she may be rushed back to the hospital that very night in real labor. These "false alarms" are a frequent source of disappointment and even of chagrin to the expectant mother, but they must be faced with equanimity since there is little to be done about them. In general, false pains are characterized by the fact that their intensity remains stationary from the outset and shows no tendency to increase with time, while the severity of true labor pains augments from hour to hour; false pains, moreover, usually occur at irregular intervals in contrast to the clocklike rhythmicity of real labor; false labor pains are rarely intensified by walking about and may even be relieved, whereas true labor pains are ordinarily aggravated by being on the feet. While, in main, these distinguishing features are valid, there are so many exceptions that the patient must not attempt to make the differentiation herself but should notify her physician at once. If any type of painful uterine contractions is associated with a discharge of bloody mucus or of water from the vagina, it is almost certain that real labor is setting in or about to set in.

In the majority of cases labor starts by intermittent, painful contractions of the uterus, but not infrequently this is preceded (and often accompanied) by the discharge of a slight amount of blood-tinged mucus. During pregnancy the neck of the uterus is closed by a thick plug of mucus. Since, as we shall see, the process of labor entails the dilatation of this canal, the plug is usually loosened and dislodged at the onset of labor and escapes through the vagina together with a drop or two of bright red blood. This phenomenon is often referred to as "show." Almost without exception, labor pains ensue within twenty-four hours after the appearance of "show."

Occasionally labor is initiated by rupture of the bag of waters. This may be followed by a sudden gush of water from the vagina or only by a slow leakage. Although this event is often followed by labor pains within a few hours, do not wait for labor pains to call the doctor as he will want to know at once if the membranes have ruptured. In the event the bag of waters should break when you are downtown or some distance away from home, it is judicious to take a taxi direct to the hospital, asking one of the hospital nurses or doctors to notify your medical attendant. Your husband can bring your grip later. These instructions, although they may suggest that rupture of the membranes is a serious occurrence, are given simply for the purpose of getting you to bed as soon as conviently possible. Rupture of the bag of waters is not a serious event and a vast number of perfectly normal and "easy" labors start in this manner.

Although it is commonly thought that most labors start at night, statistics show that the times of onset, as well as the times of actual birth, are rather evenly distributed around the clock. For instance, the late Dr. Joseph B. De Lee reported that in 1000 confinements at the Chicago Lying-in Hospital, labor began and ended as follows:

Labor began		*Labor ended*
274	Between 6 P.M. and midnight	229
306	Between midnight and 6 A.M.	278
238	Between 6 A.M. and noon	267
182	Between noon and 6 P.M.	226

Accordingly, while there seems to be a slightly greater likelihood of labor's starting and ending at night, rather than in the day, the tendency is not striking. It may be well to note, however, that the chances of labor's *either* starting *or* ending at night are excellent.

When to Call the Doctor. — In general, the doctor should be notified just as soon as you think you are in labor, as evidenced by the signs just reviewed. If this is the first baby, an hour or so of regularly recurrent pains, fifteen minutes apart, which tend to increase in severity is usually sufficient evidence. Women who have had previous children and who are therefore better able to recognize and evaluate labor pains may find it desirable to call in less than an hour, depending upon the severity of the pains, their frequency and the patient's experience in previous confinements. As we have already indicated, any type of painful uterine contraction when associated with "show" is strong evidence that labor is starting, and, as just emphasized, rupture of the membranes, with or without pains, demands immediate notification of the doctor. If in doubt, err on the side of calling the doctor and ask his advice.

"Overdue" Babies. — As we have previously stated (pages 38-40), the likelihood that you will start in labor on the exact day calculated for your confinement is small; and the chances are one in ten, let us remember, that you will go two weeks beyond that date. This is always a trying, irksome period, beset by "false alarms," no doubt, and by sundry discomforts — to say nothing of daily calls from solicitous friends inquiring whether pregnancy is to be your chronic state. As a result, not a few expectant mothers become impatient and want something done to initiate labor. Unfortunately, such a step is not always in the best interests of yourself and the baby; and in the long run, it is usually wiser to exhaust your patience still further and wait. Very few babies are actually "overdue"; they just seem to be because unwarranted reliance has been put on the calculated date, which, as we have shown, is merely a rough guess.

Now and then, however, circumstances arise in which your doctor, after weighing all aspects of the case, may recommend that labor be induced. Perhaps the first attempt will be made by the well-known expedient of castor oil, with or without a small dose of quinine, followed by a hot soapsuds enema. The easiest way to take castor oil is as follows: After coating the inner surface and edges of a drinking glass with orange juice, pour in a few tablespoonfuls of the orange juice, then the castor oil and finally a few more tablespoonfuls of orange juice on top. Now comes the most important part. Place in your mouth, well back against the palate, a piece of ice about the size of a walnut and hold it there until it becomes quite painful; this temporarily paralyzes the taste buds on the tongue, and if the "sandwich" of castor oil and orange juice is taken as soon as the ice is removed, there is little or no sense of taste. Although this method of inducing labor is sometimes referred to as harmless, it should never be employed, of course, without the recommendation of your physician, who will specify the dosage and other details.

Even in women who are at or beyond their expected date of confinement, the castor-oil program fails rather more often than it succeeds; so prepare for disappoint-ment. Other methods of inducing labor, sometimes used in association with castor oil, sometimes alone, are hypo-dermic injections of pituitrin (a uterine stimulant) in minute doses; the application of the same drug to the interior of the nose whence it is absorbed; and artificial puncture of the bag of waters. The latter procedure not infrequently necessitates a few minutes of anesthesia. Provided that conditions are favorable, puncture of the bag of waters is almost always followed by labor within a few hours; but it is a procedure which should be done only when your doctor has sound reasons for it.

Admission to the Hospital. — Many women have a dread of not getting to the hospital in time. Such fears are based largely on occasional newspaper reports of ba-bies' being born in taxicabs, on the front steps of hospi-tals and in other unorthodox places. It is true that this happens now and then, but the very fact that such an event is seized upon so avidly by the press is proof enough of its rarity. Provided that ordinary common sense is used in asking the doctor's advice as soon as labor seems to have begun, there is no great rush about getting to the hospital and the trip should be made leisurely. The doc-tor will have notified the institution and everything will be in readiness for you.

For many a young woman, admission to a maternity ward marks her first acquaintance with hospitals, as well as with the world of nurses and doctors. The immediate reaction may be one of strangeness, of loneliness and of homesickness. The nurses, in their stiff, white uniforms, may seem on first acquaintance somewhat stern and forbidding; you may even chronicle the impression that, to them, you are just another "case," which they are handling in a very matter-of-fact and routine sort of way. But beware of first impressions. Beneath their starched and sedate exteriors, these daughters of Florence Nightingale cherish but one mission in life, the safety of such as you and yours; your welfare and that of your baby are their greatest concern and their greatest pride; let either of you show the slightest deviation from normal, and they are at attention to raise heaven and earth in your behalf. If they seem businesslike, it is only because of their earnest desire to carry out every detail of the care necessary for your well-being. And what about the hospital doctors, the young men in white who venture hesitatingly into your room at odd moments, ask all kinds of silly questions and insist on thumping your chest or getting a drop of blood from your finger? Much maligned are these young men by misunderstanding patients, and a word in their support seems in order. They are doctors of medicine, you understand, who have gone through the most arduous period of study and training known to any of the learned professions. As medical students they have conducted dozens of deliveries and assisted at scores more; and they have passed no end of exacting examinations in obstetrics and every other branch of medicine. This may be their first, second, or even their third year out of school. Fresh from training in the latest scientific methods, they have at their finger tips an array of procedures which may be of the utmost help to your own physician, who will rely on them for much valuable assistance. The presence of interns and residents in hospitals makes it possible for you to have the benefit of two medical attendants: your own private doctor, mature in judgment and experienced; and, as an assistant, a younger hospital physician whose special skill in certain minutiae of diagnosis and treatment makes him invaluable. Both are essential if the very finest type of medical care is to be given.

Preliminary Preparations for Delivery. — After it is definitely established that labor is under way, the nurse carries out certain preliminary preparations for delivery, the exact nature of which will depend on the wishes of the doctor and the custom of the particular hospital. The nurse assists the patient to undress, helps her into a hospital gown and sees that she is comfortable in bed. In many instances the doctor will wish an enema given, in others, not; in case this is administered, a bedpan will be employed since it is inadvisable to use the toilet at this time. As a rule, the chief procedure in preparing for delivery is shaving the region over the pubic bone and about the vaginal orifice; in some institutions, clipping of the hair is done, instead. Then, with the nurse in assistance, the doctor, possibly your own doctor, possibly the hospital physician, examines the blood pressure, heart and chest; a checking up on the latter is particularly necessary in order to make sure that there is no evidence of a recent cold or bronchitis, findings which would have a bearing on the type of anesthesia used when the baby is born. The abdominal examinations carried out at this time are the same as those made during the prenatal period, and are simply a survey to ascertain that the baby is in good position and its heart sounds audible. The nurse now drapes a sheet about the legs and thighs of the patient in preparation for an internal examination which is of the utmost importance to make certain that labor is progressing normally. This may be done by either the rectal or the vaginal route. No particular preparation is necessary for a rectal examination; the doctor merely slips his gloved forefinger into the rectum to determine the position of the baby's head and the degree of widening which the birth canal is undergoing. In the event a vaginal examination is made, the nurse carefully cleanses the region about the vaginal orifice with antiseptic fluids, while the doctor submits his hands to prolonged scrubbing and dons a sterile rubber glove. As stated previously, these internal examinations are not disturbing if the patient will relax completely. They are usually repeated from time to time during the course of labor.

What Happens in Labor. — Reduced to its simplest constituents, the process of labor resolves itself into the expulsion from the uterus of the products of conception, that is, the baby, afterbirth, membranes and fluid. As may be seen in Figure 7, the lower portion of the uterus converges into a spindle-shaped structure, the neck of the uterus, or as doctors call it, the cervix. Running through the cervix is a slender canal, a canal which serves in the nonpregnant state for the escape of menstrual blood. Since it is through this same channel that the baby must pass, it is obvious that the neck of the uterus must dilate greatly as a preliminary to the expulsion of the infant. From the viewpoint of the time involved, the greater part of labor is devoted to this di-

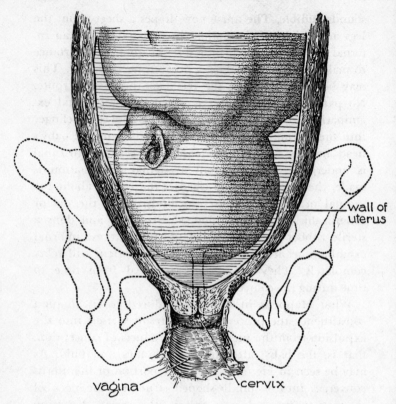

Figure 7. Condition of the Cervix (Neck of the Uterus) before Labor Sets In. Bag of Waters Intact.

lating stage, or, as it is called in medical terminology, the "first stage of labor." During this period the contractions of the uterus exert pressure on the baby and bag of waters, forcing them gradually downward and into the cervix; by this means, little by little, dilatation of the canal is brought about. (Figures 8 and 9.)

At the beginning of the dilating stage of labor the pains are mild and, as we have said, occur at intervals of fifteen or twenty minutes; but they gradually increase in severity and after a few hours recur every four or five minutes. Between pains, as a rule, the patient is entirely comfortable. If the pains become exceedingly severe, it is usually possible for the doctor to administer some pain-relieving drug, a subject which will be discussed in the next chapter. During this period an effort should be made to relax as much as possible and to rest between pains; no attempt should be made to "bear down," that is, to contract the abdominal muscles in an expulsive effort such as is employed when the bowels move. This is futile at this time and merely uses up strength unnecessarily. Toward the end of the dilating stage, the bag of waters very often ruptures and the patient becomes aware of the escape of fluid.

The second stage of labor begins when the cervix is fully dilated (about four inches in diameter) and ends with the birth of the child; since it is concerned with the expelling of the infant, it is often called the "stage of expulsion." This stage is much shorter than the first stage, averaging something over an hour and a half with first babies and about thirty minutes with subsequent children. Sometimes, anesthesia is given with each pain throughout the greater part or all of this period. It must be remembered that the expulsion of the infant is brought about by the action of the abdominal and respiratory muscles in much the same way as a bowel move-

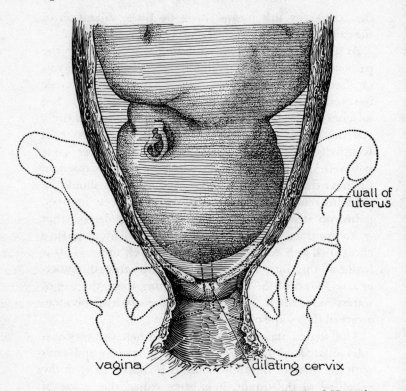

wall of
uterus

vagina dilating cervix

Figure 8. Beginning of Dilatation of Cervix (Neck of Uterus).
Bag of Waters Still Intact.

ment is accomplished. Accordingly, at this stage of labor, the patient may be asked to exert these muscular forces and bear down with each pain. A common practice is as follows: the moment the patient feels a pain coming on (there are several seconds of warning), she takes three or four deep whiffs of the anesthetic (usually ni-

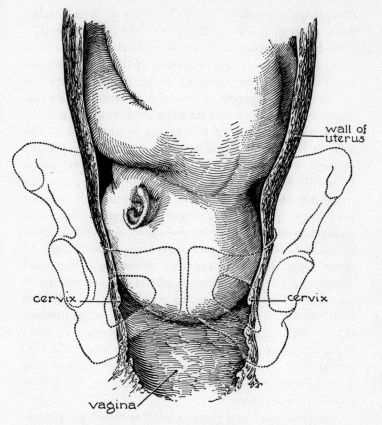

Figure 9. Complete Dilatation of the Cervix (Neck of Uterus).
The Bag of Waters Has Ruptured and the Head Has
Descended to a Lower Level.

trous oxide — "laughing gas"), closes her lips, holds her
breath and strains down. Meanwhile, the anesthetic has
taken effect and she carries out the desired procedure al-

though unconscious of it. With each pain and bearing down effort of this kind, the head of the baby descends a little farther, finally distends the vaginal opening and is born; the shoulders and remainder of the body then follow rapidly. As the moment of birth approaches, the anesthesia is deepened so that the patient is quite unconscious at this time and for a few minutes afterward.

The degree to which the vagina is distended as the baby is born is a source of dismay to many expectant mothers who fancy that deep tears must be inevitable. It is true that the vagina of the nonpregnant woman could not be stretched to any such extent. Throughout pregnancy, however, the vagina undergoes progressive changes in the way of increased succulence and distensibility and toward the end may easily be stretched to many times its former capacity. Accordingly, the tears which do occur are usually superficial and are readily repaired by a few stitches which are taken while the mother is still under the anesthesia. Some doctors, when they see that a tear is inevitable, forestall its occurrence by making a small cut with scissors at the place where the tear would have occurred, thus substituting for a jagged tear a straight surgical incision, which heals better; this is called an "episiotomy."

The third and final stage of labor is called the placental stage since it has to do with the expulsion of the afterbirth. It rarely lasts longer than fifteen minutes and is associated with little or no pain. As a rule, the doctor assists the passage of the placenta by gentle pressure over the pubic bone. After the birth of the placenta a certain amount of bleeding is normal, the quantity of blood lost averaging slightly more than half a pint. In order that the bleeding may not become excessive, a uterine stimulant is frequently given by hypodermic and the uterus, now a hard, globular mass just below the navel, may be massaged. These measures cause the interlacing muscle fibers of the uterus to contract so tightly that the blood vessels in their interstices are squeezed shut and further bleeding stopped.

Duration of Labor. — The length of labor varies so greatly that it is impossible to predict in a given case how long it will last. Even when labor is well under way, prophecies as to when birth will occur are of little value, since the duration of the process depends chiefly on factors which cannot be foretold, namely, the frequency and strength of the labor pains. The average duration of labor with first babies approximates sixteen hours and with subsequent children ten hours. The longer duration of labor in first confinements results, of course, from the fact that the neck of the uterus, as well as the vagina, is more tense and unyielding; once these structures have been stretched by the birth of a child, they never again offer as much resistance to dilatation as at the first labor. Even in women having their first baby, labors under three hours occur now and then, possibly once in a hundred cases; in later confinements, such rapid, or "precipitate," labors are rather common, being seen as often as once in fifteen cases, perhaps. Labors which exceed twenty-four hours are usually due to the fact that the pains are infrequent, of short duration and weak. In other words, here is a circumstance in which certain muscular forces have a definite task to perform, that is, dilatation of the neck of the uterus and expulsion of the baby. In some women these forces act vigorously and at frequent intervals so that the task is completed rapidly; in some, they act in a more leisurely fashion and hence the undertaking requires longer. Other things being equal, labors of five hours and of twenty hours are equally normal and the outcome equally happy.

Contrary to general opinion, age has little bearing on the duration of labor, a fact of especial interest in these days when many women marry relatively late in life. The course of first labors in women over thirty-five has been the object of particular study and the evidence is clear that only a slight increase in length occurs; some statistics indicate that the average duration of such labors may be an hour and a half longer, others that it may be as much as four hours longer, but the difference is certainly not great; in one large series of cases, 20 per cent of the women had strikingly rapid and easy labor. Nor is the incidence of complications greatly higher in this older age group. Accordingly, there is no reason for the woman of thirty-five, or even of forty, to be deterred from childbirth merely by reason of age.

Forceps Delivery. — In the early decades of the seventeenth century, a new and mysterious force was making itself felt in childbirth. It became known in London that in case a woman was experiencing a prolonged labor, delivery could be effected with incredible despatch if any member of a certain family of physicians was called in and allowed to take charge. The name of the family was Chamberlen. One of the Doctors Chamberlen would appear with a bundle beneath his coat and proceed to hasten delivery under cover of a large sheet or blanket so that no one could see what he was doing; a great clanking of metal would be heard and forthwith the baby would be handed out from beneath the covers. Some more clanking of metal would occur and then Dr. Chamberlen, with his bundle carefully concealed under his coat, would be ready to collect his fee and depart. As a result of the metallic noises heard, and probably also because of the temporary marks which were sometimes left on the baby's head, the device by which the Doctors Chamberlen effected delivery became known as the "Hands of Iron"; and this was all that was known. For three generations — over a hundred years — this family of Chamberlens kept secret the instrument which has done more to abridge human suffering and to save human life than any other device in the whole range of surgical appliances. The "Hands of Iron," of course, were the obstetrical forceps.

The modern obstetrical forceps consist of two separate blades with smooth inner surfaces curved to fit the sides of the baby's head. After the patient has been completely anesthetized, the blades are inserted separately, first the left and then the right; they are next crossed and fitted together by an articulating device in such a manner that a gentle but firm grasp is obtained on the baby's head, which is then slowly extracted by means of moderate traction on the blades.

"Taking the baby with instruments" used to be regarded as an ominous procedure by the laity and the term still has a fearsome ring to many expectant parents. Today, the operation is carried out under such different conditions than formerly that it is almost a different procedure and warrants little concern. Nowadays, the majority of forceps deliveries are performed when the baby's head is almost ready to be born and are done merely to relieve the patient of the last fifteen or twenty minutes of labor; the head is simply "lifted out," as it were, instead of being pushed out by the expulsive efforts of the mother. Whether it is best to expedite delivery in this manner depends upon the circumstances presented by the individual case and will be decided, of course, by the physician. Forceps are often used for other reasons; but the most important fact for the expectant mother and members of the family to know about these instruments is that they can be used safely only toward the end of labor, when the cervix has been fully dilated and when certain other prerequisite conditions are present. In view of this fact, the doctor should never be urged to "take the baby"; he alone is in a position to understand whether these prerequisites have been fulfilled and to know when forceps delivery is an advantageous procedure and when it is not.

Cesarean Section. — The operation of cesarean section comprises cutting through the abdominal wall and uterus and removing the child through the incisions thus made; both incisions are then carefully repaired by stitches. During the past quarter of a century the incidence of cesarean section in this country has increased more than fivefold and today approximately one American baby in fifty is delivered by this means. So common has the operation become that a number of women have gained the impression that this is the easiest way of having a baby and even ask the doctor if it is not possible for them to be delivered in this fashion. Such implicit faith in cesarean section is based on misinformation. Although it is true that modern surgical methods have greatly reduced the seriousness of the procedure, it is not as safe for the mother as normal delivery through the birth canal; cesarean section is a major abdominal operation and such operative procedures are always associated with a certain small risk which is somewhat greater than that of ordinary childbirth. Another objection to cesarean section is that the woman is left a sort of cripple in so far as future childbearing is concerned: that is, because of the scar in the uterus, it is often necessary for her to be delivered by cesarean section in all later confinements. A number of authorities, it is true, take a different viewpoint and allow vaginal delivery after cesarean section. It is, nevertheless, obligatory that every woman who has had a previous cesarean section be in the hands of an obstetrical specialist throughout any subsequent pregnancy and be delivered in a hospital.

Although cesarean section is more dangerous to the mother than *normal* childbirth, it is often safer than vaginal delivery in the presence of certain complications. Childbirth, it will be recalled, consists in the passage of the baby through a bony birth canal, the pelvis. Now, if the pelvis is unusually small, the baby's transit may conceivably be impeded; and under such circumstances, cesarean section may be recommended by your physician. Certain other conditions also justify the use of the operation occasionally, but as we have indicated, forty-nine women out of fifty can be delivered by the vaginal route without appreciable difficulty.

Breech Position. — In about 96 per cent of all cases the head of the baby is born first, but in 3 per cent, approximately, the buttocks of the infant enter the pelvis and, together with the legs, are the first parts to be delivered; in the latter instance, the baby is said to be in "breech position." Although a baby may be in breech position during the greater part of pregnancy, it frequently changes its position, as the time of confinement approaches, the head entering the pelvis before labor starts. Breech positions carry a slightly greater risk to the infant, but in nine cases out of ten, the outcome is entirely satisfactory. In so far as the mother is concerned, breech labors differ very little from those in which the head is born first.

Chapter IX

"PAINLESS CHILDBIRTH"

. . . Not poppy, nor mandragora,
Nor all the drowsy syrups of the world,
Shall ever medicine thee to that sweet sleep.

SHAKESPEARE: *Othello*

THE crusade against pain in childbirth, concerning which we read so much in women's magazines today, is not new but represents the culmination of a campaign which is more than a century old. It may be said to have started late on the evening of November 4, 1847, in the dining room of a house at 52 Queen Street, Edinburgh, Scotland. Three men sat huddled over as many glass tumblers on the dining-room table. One of the group — a big-headed, shaggy-haired man whose black eyes sparkled with enthusiasm — was busy with a series of evil-smelling bottles. As if to sample the contents of each bottle, he would pour a small quantity from each, one by one, into the tumblers. From all outward appearances, this might well have been a wine-sampling party, or a search after the elixir of youth. But all the men did was to bend over the glasses, as each was newly charged, and inhale deeply. For many evenings this same curious performance had been going on, but inhale what they might, nothing happened. It was not until this particular evening, when a particular, rather sweet-smelling sub-stance was placed before them, that their quest was finally satisfied. With the first whiff of this chemical, an unwonted gaiety seized the group; with the second, an overwhelming sleepiness befell them; and scarcely had they taken the third inhalation when the three lay sprawling on the floor, not to awaken for two or three minutes. It was in this quaint fashion, over his dining-room table in Edinburgh, that Sir James Y. Simpson, to-gether with two friends, discovered the anesthetic value of chloroform. And to this day, every mother is the debtor of this great Scotch doctor, for his chief purpose in thus seeking a new anesthetic was to relieve pain in childbirth.

But Simpson faced a stubborn, uphill fight, for no sooner had he announced that the pains of childbirth could be relieved by chloroform than a storm of invec-tive befell him, from the clergy and the public, as well as from many members of the medical profession. "It is unnatural thus to interfere with the pains of childbirth which are a *natural* function," they cried. "But, is not walking also a natural function?" replied Simpson. "And who would think of never setting aside or superseding this natural function? If you were traveling from Phila-delphia to Baltimore, would you insist on walking the distance on foot simply because walking is man's natural method of locomotion?" Exclaimed an Irish lady to him one day, "How unnatural it is for you doctors in Edin-burgh to take away the pains of your patients when in labor." "How unnatural," he replied, "it is for you to have swum over from Ireland to Scotland against wind and tide in a steamboat." To the clergy's objection that such anesthesia was contrary to the Bible, and the birth-pang curse of *Paradise Lost,* he cited the "first surgical operation" and the "first anesthesia": "And the Lord God caused a deep sleep to fall upon Adam; and he slept; and he took one of his ribs, and closed up the flesh instead thereof." Countless other objections were hurled at him, but to each he had an answer; he pointed out, moreover, that all things new are likely to arouse censure, particularly censure of a religious nature. Thus, he recalled, when vaccination against smallpox was introduced, various clergymen attacked the practice as irreligious, referring to it as a tempting of God's providence and therefore a heinous crime. He cited further the introduction of table forks. At first this innovation was regarded as a very sad and uncalled-for intrusion upon the old and established natural functions of the human fingers and a number of preachers denounced it "as an insult on Providence not to touch our meat with our fingers."

To anyone acquainted with the women's magazines of today, these old disputes sound very modern, for the debate over pain relief in childbirth still continues. On the one hand, we read that it is unnecessary for a woman to suffer the slightest discomfort in childbirth. Cases are described in which, almost with the first twinge of backache, the mother falls peaceably asleep with a pill or two and awakens to find the baby in her arms. The impression is given that the method is applicable in every case, never fails and is completely harmless to mother and child; and the inference is that the mother who does not receive such pain relief has been shamefully neglected by a cruel doctor. In other articles we read that the woman who accepts such medication not only misses a "soul-satisfying experience" but compromises the safety of the baby for her own comfort and is hence a cowardly and selfish creature. A few years ago these altercations were threshed out at a meeting of the American Medical Association and were wrangled over endlessly by our country's leading obstetricians. When such experts as these disagree in respect to the feasibility of "painless childbirth," it is understandable that the lay press is at odds and that the expectant mother may be hopelessly vexed in regard to this question.

What is the truth about pain relief in labor?

For the purposes of the present discussion the pain of childbirth may be divided into three phases. In the first place, there is a period of preliminary pains lasting, as a rule, several hours. These are mild in degree and are rarely disturbing; even after the pains have become sufficiently definite to warrant going to the hospital, most women are able to carry on with their reading, knitting or whatnot. These pains serve a useful purpose in warning the woman that labor is starting; indeed, if the whole process of labor were completely painless, babies would be born in the most inconvenient places. There follows a second phase, of six to ten hours' duration perhaps, in which the pains are more severe; this comprises the greater part of the dilating phase and as complete dilatation is reached, the pains usually reach their maximum. We shall return to this period presently. The third phase of pain is associated with the expulsion of the baby and lasts, as we have indicated, between twenty minutes and two hours. Today, almost without exception, some form of anesthesia is administered for the actual delivery of the baby. The type used will depend on the circumstances presented by the individual case and on the preference of the particular obstetrician. One type is inhalation anesthesia (gas-oxygen, ether, etc.); another is spinal anesthesia (page 163), which eliminates all sensation in the pelvic region; while still another is the local injection of anesthetic agents. One of the more commonly employed methods of anesthesia during the expulsive stage is nitrous oxide, or laughing gas. This is often started before complete dilatation of the cervix (when the pains are approaching their maximum) and continued until after the birth of the baby. As we have described in the previous chapter, the gas is given with each successive pain, the patient being allowed to awaken between pains. Ether is sometimes used for the same purpose but is slower in action; it is more often given in association with nitrous oxide as the birth of the baby approaches in order to deepen the anesthesia. A vast experience has shown that anesthesia with either nitrous oxide or ether, administered with pains and deepened for the actual birth of the baby, eliminates most of the pain associated with the expulsive stage. Furthermore, provided the mother is in a normal state of health and the baby has gone to full term, these measures are relatively safe for mother and child alike; with rare exceptions all doctors are in agreement on this point.

Since the preliminary pains are not severe enough to

be disturbing and since those of the expulsive stage may be easily and safely eliminated by anesthesia, the only pains which need concern us are those met in the middle part of labor, the dilating pains. It is over these that the modern controversy persists. Ether by inhalation is of no use at this time since it retards labor; nor can nitrous oxide be employed successfully throughout this stage. There are, however, a group of drugs which can be administered either by hypodermic needle, by mouth or by inhalation, some of which alleviate pain and others of which, either alone or in combination, abolish the memory of pain. Let us consider both the usefulness and the drawbacks of these drugs.

Twilight Sleep. — By "Twilight Sleep" is meant a regime in which morphine is combined with scopolamine, a drug which obliterates memory of whatever events occur when under its influence. Its aim is not so much actual pain relief as forgetfulness, or amnesia (Greek for "without memory"). Thus, a woman under Twilight Sleep may shriek, make grimaces and show other evidences of pain, but upon awakening from the drug will remember nothing about her labor and will vow that she experienced no pain whatsoever. Introduced in Germany during the early years of this century, this method met with wide acclaim in the United States about 1915, and was the subject of many feature articles in magazines. "Women of America," reads one appeal, "ask for it. Demand it. Insist upon it. Tolerate no other way . . . than Twilight Sleep." Then, as now, ill-informed feature writers expatiated in this extravagant fashion about painless childbirth without appreciating the whole truth. They were not in a position to know, as physicians did, that Twilight Sleep imposed a slight but definite handicap on the baby's ability to breathe at birth, and was particularly detrimental to certain very small babies. The original Twilight Sleep is still used successfully by a number of physicians, but its administration requires the utmost care and judgment. From a historical point of view, the introduction of Twilight Sleep was of immense importance, for it focused attention on the possibilities of amnesia in childbirth and pointed the way to some of our more modern and safer methods.

Barbiturates. — By barbiturates we mean a group of sleep-producing drugs derived from a mother substance, barbituric acid; Luminal, barbital, sodium Amytal, Seconal and Nembutal are a few of the drugs belonging to this group. They may be given alone or in combination with scopolamine. The general effect is similar to that of Twilight Sleep, that is, pain relief plus amnesia. The results are usually very satisfactory, the patient knowing nothing about her labor and awakening in her own room several hours after the baby has been born. It is true that these drugs exert a slightly depressing effect on the baby, but statistics indicate that normal, full-term babies do just as well under this regime as they do in cases in which no sedatives were used in the dilating stage.

Demerol. — Demerol is another drug which is extensively used to produce sedation and, when combined with scopolamine, provides amnesia also. Although not a barbiturate but a morphine derivative, its effects resemble somewhat those of the barbiturates and it is preferred by many doctors.

Although drugs such as the barbiturates and Demerol, as well as inhalation anesthesia such as gas-oxygen-ether, exert little or no effect on the normal, full-term infant, they are very likely to impair the outlook for a prematurely born baby because its incompletely developed respiratory system is especially vulnerable to the depressing action of these agents. Hence, if you go into labor a month or more before your expected date of confinement, your physician may, for the sake of the baby, withhold these drugs and use some other method of pain relief even if less efficacious.

Trilene. — Trilene is an anesthetic liquid which resembles chloroform in smell and effects. It is *self-administered* by means of an inhaler which consists of a mask and an adjoining compartment containing the Trilene. Trilene evaporates readily at room temperature, and by putting the mask over her face the patient can inhale the Trilene vapor with each labor pain as she may desire. The inhaler is attached to the mother's wrist by a strap so that the inhaler automatically falls from her face the moment unconsciousness is reached. The patient regains complete consciousness between pains.

Trilene provides a safe pain relief and most patients find it very helpful. Although some women object to the odor of Trilene at first, they rapidly become accustomed to it after the vapor has been inhaled a few times. The attitude of doctors toward Trilene varies. Many endorse it but the majority prefer other techniques on the grounds that they are more efficacious.

Spinal and Continuous Caudal Anesthesia. — It is one of the functions of the vertebral column or backbone — which is essentially a bony tube — to house the nerves along which impulses run back and forth between the brain and various parts of the body. A substantial portion of these nerves convey to the brain the various sensations received, such as the feeling of cold, heat or pain. If any of these nerves is benumbed by the application of an anesthetic drug, it is no longer able to convey impulses and hence no sensations are received by the brain from the part of the body supplied by the particular nerve or nerves anesthetized. This is the basis of both spinal and caudal anesthesia, since both entail introducing an anesthetic solution into the interior spaces of the vertebral column where the drug bathes these nerves and temporarily deadens them. In both of these forms of anesthesia the patient is entirely conscious, but is oblivious to pain or other sensations from the uterus or birth canal.

In spinal anesthesia the drug is introduced directly into the spinal canal in the region of the small of the back. It is employed chiefly for actual delivery but is sometimes used to cover the last few hours of labor. In caudal anesthesia the drug is introduced somewhat lower and into a bony space at the very lower end of the vertebral column. By renewing this anesthetic solution from time to time, as its effects wear off, it is possible to make caudal anesthesia "continuous" for as long as six or eight hours, sometimes longer.

When this continuous caudal anesthesia was first introduced in 1942, it was received with wide acclaim by popular magazines and everyone hoped it was the long-sought, ideal method of eliminating pain in every labor. Time and experience have shown, however, that these early hopes were not justified and that it is suitable and efficacious only in certain cases; and then it has its drawbacks as well as its advantages.

Local Anesthesia. — By injecting a solution containing an appropriate anesthetic drug into the regions surrounding the vagina, the nerves which supply that area are blocked and the entire region is made insensitive to pain. Because of its high degree of safety this method has gained wide popularity and is employed especially for "lifting the baby out" with forceps, as explained on pages 150-152.

*   *   *   *

Since any of the drugs mentioned above may be used either alone, or in combination with any of the others listed, it is apparent that various regimes are available for the relief of the dilating pains of labor. Now, whenever a large number of different remedies are in use for the treatment of a given condition, the chances are that no single one is entirely satisfactory. And this is very true of these drugs employed in childbirth. None are without their drawbacks; none are applicable in all cases; and none are without some slight risk to the mother or child under certain circumstances. Moreover, with a few exceptions, none can be employed except in hospitals with a special nurse in constant attendance. It is for these several reasons that a certain section of medical opinion questions the wisdom of using them. In passing, it may be noted that it is for these same reasons that the decision in regard to pain relief must rest entirely with the doctor, who alone is in a position to know when these agents are completely safe and when they are not.

On the other side of the question, the number of women who are enjoying practically painless labors is mounting annually. Statistics show clearly that when good medical judgment is exercised in their employment, these drugs yield results to both mother and child which are excellent. Doctors who specialize in maternity work pride themselves on the large proportion of their patients who have only pleasant memories of their labors; and in the immediate future still further improvement is certain to ensue, for a whole army of workers is bent on finding new and more efficacious procedures.

Accordingly, the expectant mother of today may face the pains of childbirth with equanimity, even with nonchalance. As we have said, the most severe pains, those of the expulsive stage, are almost always eliminated by anesthesia, while those of the dilating period are usually met in one of the ways described. Indeed, you need have no more fear of labor pains than of those of the dentist chair and should follow a similar policy in dealing with both situations. In other words, if the pains become unbearably severe, you should so inform the doctor. In all probability he will be able to lessen their intensity at once; and perhaps he will send you off with a magic pill to some distant country of dreams.

Natural Childbirth. — Publicity about Natural Childbirth in the press and magazines has advanced so many misconceptions about it that it has come to mean many erroneous things to many people. First, let us correct one widespread notion: it does not mean "painless childbirth." Even the most enthusiastic adherents of Natural Childbirth do not claim that it yields painless labors. Only drugs can do that. Nor does it necessarily mean "drugless labors," because medication is used in a substantial number of cases, although in lower dosage perhaps than would otherwise have been employed.

In essence, Natural Childbirth represents an attempt to make labor easier through the elimination of fear. It is based on the premise that labors are easier in women who are placid, worry-free and relaxed. This is undoubtedly true; but how can this placid, worry-free and relaxed state be achieved? In three ways, as follows:

The transcendent prerequisite is that you have complete confidence in your doctor — confidence that he is your friend, a medically wise friend who is sincerely desirous of sparing you all the pain possible, provided that this is compatible with your welfare and that of your child. The very presence of such a friendly doctor, and the realization that he is competent to handle any situation, is in itself the most effective and welcome of obstetric anodynes.

In the second place, acquaint yourself with the natural, physiologic changes which will take place in your body as pregnancy advances so that you may know what to expect. Learn also what will transpire in labor, including what the doctors and the nurses will do, so that nothing will be new, unexpected or strange. It is the purpose of this book to provide such information.

Finally, learn to relax, let yourself go loose and take it easy. Moreover, remember to do this in labor.

If you will but do these three things you will secure all the advantages of Natural Childbirth and need not bother further about it. Actually, all good doctors have been following the main tenets of Natural Childbirth for years.

Some women, either through curiosity or for other reasons, request that they receive no medication whatsoever for pain in labor. This is well and good; and most doctors will be happy to abide by such requests and give all the encouragement possible. But if you fall in this group and subsequently change your mind in favor of a sedative, do not feel therefore that you have been a complete disgrace to womanhood. Indeed, provided your doctor thinks that medication is desirable, there is no more sense or glory in a "do-or-die" determination to go through labor without pain relief than there would be to refuse anesthesia for a tooth extraction.

Chapter X

CONVALESCENCE FROM CHILDBIRTH

A PERIOD of six to eight weeks is required after childbirth for the uterus and other pelvic structures to return to their former condition. This interval is referred to by physicians as the "puerperium," a term derived from the Latin words *puer,* a child, and *pario,* to bear. By and large, the puerperium should be a happy and pleasant experience. The majority of women feel quite well throughout this period. As a rule, the discomforts are few in number and minor in character; and, to offset them, there is the long-awaited baby, to say nothing of the fact that at last your abdomen is flat — to most women an almost unbelievable achievement! At the same time, from the viewpoint of mother and child alike, this period of convalescence is of far-reaching importance since the future health of both depends on proper rest and care during these weeks.

In most instances, the mother's first experience in the puerperium is awakening from the anesthetic to find the hand of a doctor or nurse exerting pressure on her lower abdomen; actually, the hand is holding her uterus and perhaps massaging it gently from time to time. The uterus, now emptied of its contents, is the size of a large grapefruit and reaches from the pubic bone to the level of the navel. The purpose of holding or massaging it at this time is to make sure that its muscle fibers remain tightly contracted so that the amount of bleeding is minimal. Accordingly, it is customary for a doctor or nurse to keep a hand on the uterus for one hour after delivery. At the end of this period the patient is usually ready to be returned to her room — and is also ready, as a rule, for a good rest.

During the following weeks two remarkable changes take place in the mother's body: the uterus retrogresses to its former size (involution) and milk develops in the breasts (lactation). Since most of the phenomena which occur in the puerperium are contingent upon these changes, let us consider them in some detail.

INVOLUTION OF UTERUS

Meaning of Involution. — The uterus, it will be recalled, has served a number of important purposes: it has given shelter to the infant for nine months, and through the placenta, has also provided its nourishment; and finally, by means of its muscular contractions, it has effected the expulsion of the baby into the outside world. Now, with its functions temporarily at an end, this structure enacts the most remarkable "disappearing feat" known to bodily economy. Within the short space of six weeks, it shrinks from an organ of two pounds to one of less than two ounces. Immediately after delivery its bulk gives a distinct bulge to the lower abdomen: within a week its weight has diminished by one half; within ten days it is usually so small that it lies entirely in the pelvic cavity and can no longer be felt through the abdominal wall. This shriveling process, by which the uterus decreases twentyfold in some six weeks, is called "involution" and is brought about by shrinkage of the individual muscle cells followed by absorption of the greater part of their contents into the general circulation.

The Lochia. — To the patient, the most noticeable phase of involution is that in which the thickened lining of the uterus (originally prepared for the embedding of the ovum) breaks down and is cast off. This gives rise to a profuse vaginal discharge, known to physicians as "the lochia." During the first four or five days of the puerperium, the discharge contains substantial amounts of blood, admixed with cast-off cellular debris, and is consequently red in color. Toward the end of the first week, the color fades to a brown; by the tenth day it has become paler, being either yellow or whitish; and finally, at the end of two or three weeks, the discharge disappears almost entirely in most cases. The amount of the lochia averages about one pint, three fourths of which is discharged in the first four days; expressed in different terms, the lochia require the use of about six pads a day during the greater part of the first week. (These pads are always furnished by the hospital.) The odor of the lochia resembles that of menstrual blood.

While the above description of the lochia holds true for the average patient, great individual variation occurs in perfectly normal cases. Now and then, without apparent cause, the red lochia will continue for a fortnight; or they may reappear after several weeks on the occasion

of excessive exertion. Indeed, the flow may continue off
and on in small amounts for as long as four weeks. Although this prolongation of bloody lochia, or their reap-
pearance, may be quite normal, such a course of events
is often an indication that the mother is overdoing and
needs more rest. If the red lochia continue after four
weeks or if, at any time after two weeks, they are as profuse as the first day of a menstrual period, the fact
should be reported to your physician.

LACTATION

Time Relationships. — In our review of the embedding
of the ovum (pages 29-30), we had occasion to remark
on the precision of the time relationships involved. In
considering the onset of lactation, or milk secretion, we
find another example of this miraculous and beneficent
timing. Although the breasts have been undergoing obvious preparatory changes throughout pregnancy, including
the secretion of colostrum (page 6), no actual milk has
been secreted; nor will any milk be secreted until after the
baby is born. Regardless of whether the baby arrives a
month prematurely, or a fortnight later than scheduled,
the onset of lactation invariably occurs at the same time
and at the right time, namely, three days after delivery,
when the baby has had time to recover from its trip
through the birth canal and is ready for food. Just how
Nature manages this schedule has long been a secret and
only recently have scientists gleaned some understanding
of the underlying mechanism. It would now appear that
the placenta, by means of certain chemical messengers sent

to various parts of the body, has the power of inhibiting or withholding the secretion of milk. Of course, when the baby is born, the placenta is also delivered, and when the inhibitory action of the placenta is removed, milk secretion gets under way.

Onset of Lactation. — Although milk usually comes into the breasts about the third day after delivery, it sometimes appears slightly later than this with first babies, and somewhat earlier with subsequent children. The event is heralded by the breasts becoming harder, fuller and heavier; the skin over them becomes tense, while the underlying veins become engorged with blood and appear swollen and distinct beneath the skin. If the baby is now put to the nipple a quantity of milk runs out. This fluid is quite different from the colostrum which has been secreted up to now, being white, opaque and very rich in sugar.

The fullness of the breasts on the day the milk comes in may cause moderate discomfort, particularly in the case of first babies. This condition is not due to an in- rush of milk, but to the congestion in the surrounding blood vessels when the milk glands begin to function. This congestion is temporary, rarely lasts longer than forty-eight hours and may be greatly relieved by a sup- portive brassière and ice packs. Once the initial conges- tion is over, the breasts become softer and more com- fortable.

Quantity of Milk. — The quantity of milk secreted in twenty-four hours varies considerably from day to day, and from mother to mother. It has been estimated, how- ever, that the average amount secreted at first is about one half pint daily; by the seventh day this has increased to almost a pint, while after the second week the quantity ranges from one pint to two pints or more.

A number of factors are known to affect the amount of milk which a woman is able to secrete and two of these every mother should be cognizant of. In the first place, nervous, worried, high-strung women usually have less milk than the happy-go-lucky type. Paradoxically enough, it is often the woman who is most solicitous and concerned about having adequate milk for her baby who has the least. In other words, if you want to nurse your baby, the more you can cultivate a carefree, worry-free attitude, the more successful you will be. Second, a large intake of fluids, particularly cow's milk, unquestionably stimulates milk production. Accordingly, a concerted effort should be made to increase the amount of water and milk consumed, making sure that the total quantity of fluids taken never falls below three quarts a day.

Quality of Milk. — Extensive investigations show that the quality of human milk varies little, provided the quantity is adequate. Nevertheless, certain extraneous factors may occasionally affect this. For instance, almost all drugs taken by the mother reappear in the milk. In the case of cathartics this has been known since the time of the ancient Greek physicians. Alcohol passes readily into the milk and several cases are on record in which the baby became intoxicated after excessive drinking by the mother. Nicotine appears in the milk of mothers who smoke, but the amounts are so small as to be of no concern. Again, there is a widespread belief that certain foods, such as tomatoes and pickles, affect the milk adversely and give the baby colic. Although medical opinion has long been skeptical of this fact, the author is convinced, on the basis of many intelligent mothers' statements, that it contains some truth. However, he does not caution the mother against any foods, but merely suggests that if repeated trials show that certain articles of diet seem to disagree with the baby, it is only common sense to avoid them.

Time of Nursing. — Doctors pursue different practices in regard to the time at which nursing is started and also in regard to the frequency of feeding during the first two or three days. Some physicians start the baby on the breast twelve hours after delivery, others twenty-four hours afterward; some begin at once with a four-hour schedule, others prefer a six-hour interval until the milk comes in. After lactation has once begun, it is common practice to bring the baby to the breast every four hours, for example, at 6 A.M., 10 A.M., 2 P.M., 6 P.M., 10 P.M., and 2 A.M. Here again custom varies and, particularly with small babies, some physicians prefer three-hour feedings during the day with one night feeding, for example, 6 A.M., 9 A.M., 12 Noon, 3 P.M., 6 P.M., 9 P.M., and 2 A.M. If the four-hour interval is employed, both breasts are nursed for ten minutes each, as a rule. With the three-hour interval, it is customary to use alternate breasts at each feeding, the duration of nursing being extended slightly. From a medical viewpoint, each of these schedules possesses advantages under certain circumstances and your physician will naturally put your baby on the schedule best suited to his particular needs.

Care of the Nipples. — Meticulous care should be exercised to keep the nipples clean. Before feedings they are usually washed either with boric-acid solution or with sterile water, while between feedings it is customary for the mother to keep a piece of sterile gauze against the nipple, the gauze being held in place by a light binder. A nursing brassière is excellent for this purpose and is a definite help, furthermore, in preventing subsequent sagging of the breasts.

Teaching the Baby to Nurse. — Although the baby is born with an active sucking reflex, not a few babies have difficulty in co-ordinating their efforts when the nipple is first put into their mouths. This sometimes seems to be the result of overenthusiasm, the baby going at the nipple with such excited gusto that he clumsily bobs the nipple out of his mouth and then loses his temper over the whole business and starts to wail. Sometimes, since he gets only a few drops of colostrum during the first few days, the baby appears to become disgruntled over the meager fare at his new boardinghouse, and after a brief trial gives every evidence that he prefers sleep to such a futile and tantalizing procedure.

However this may be, the mother should understand that the chief purpose of putting the baby to the breast these first two days is to educate him (and also her) in the serious business of nursing. The baby should be held in such a manner that he need exercise no effort to contact the breast, that is, he should not be made to stretch his neck forward in order to reach the nipple. In so far as the mother's condition permits, the baby should be held in a semi-reclining position, rather than in a horizontal one; babies take more milk in this position and are less likely to swallow air. It should also be remembered that the baby must breathe solely through his nose while suckling and that a clear nasal pathway is essential for good nursing. If the breast is large and allowed to press against the baby's nose, his nasal pathway may be obstructed and he will gulp and swallow air in his efforts to breathe. Even with these precautions against swallowing air, X-ray studies show that an air bubble is almost invariably present in the infant's stomach after nursing. It is therefore a common practice for the mother or nurse to place the baby over her shoulder after nursing, pat him gently on the back and thus release the bubble. This is referred to as "bubbling" the baby. The nurse will be of invaluable assistance in getting suckling started since she will know a dozen or more tricks and maneuvers to accomplish the desired end. In any event, the problem involved is rarely a serious matter but merely one which occasionally requires a little patience.

Breast versus Artificial Feeding. — During recent years several articles in lay magazines have again brought this old problem to the fore. As was true of the controversy over pain relief in labor, the arguments on both sides of this question tend toward exaggeration. On the one hand, we are led to believe that artificial, or bottle, feeding, being based on modern, scientific calculations, is actually superior to the "old-fashioned method." On the other hand, we are told that the mother who fails to nurse her baby condemns it to an appalling hazard, to sundry diseases, to an ugly lower jaw and even to a faulty background in filial piety. Where does the truth lie? Should you nurse your baby? Must you nurse your baby? Let us approach the question from a common-sense point of view and try to evaluate honestly the merits and drawbacks of the two methods.

The advantages of breast-feeding are many:

1. Human milk is the ideal food for the newborn. It contains most of the substances necessary for maintenance, growth and development during the first months of life in just the correct proportion for optimal digestion and absorption. Cow's milk, it must be remembered, differs from human milk in many important respects. Thus, it contains almost two and a half times as much protein as human milk; furthermore, this protein of cow's milk, when it enters the stomach, divides into relatively large curds which are less easily digested than the fine, soft curds into which the protein of human milk is dispersed. There is likewise considerable difference in the sugar contents, human milk being very rich in this ingredient. Although the latter difficulty may be met by adding sugar to cow's milk, the fact remains that the *quality* of the ingredients of human milk makes it the most easily digestible food for the newborn infant.

2. Breast milk is normally clean; and if reasonable care is observed, the milk ingested by the baby is entirely free of harmful bacteria. Moreover, since no storing of the milk is entailed, there is no possibility of deterioration.

3. Stomach and intestinal disturbances (doubtless for the reasons just cited) are rare in breast-fed babies. Constipation is less common. In the event the stools do

manifest any irregularity (change in color, consistency, etc.), there is never cause for concern since nothing can be wrong with the food and the condition is sure to right itself; whereas, abnormalities of the stool in a bottle-fed baby often indicate that one or another ingredient in the formula is present in excess and a shift in the formula becomes necessary.

4. Nature has packed more food value (calories) per ounce in human milk than it is usually possible to introduce into a formula. Consequently, the baby receives more food, as a rule, and gains more rapidly.

5. Breast-feeding, through a curious connection between the uterus and breasts, hastens involution of the uterus so that the mother's reproductive organs return to normal more rapidly.

6. Breast-feeding is usually more convenient for the mother. There are no complicated formulas to measure out, no temperature levels to adjust and no storage problems. There are no trips to the kitchen at 6 A.M. for a bottle and no standing over the stove while it warms. Breast-feeding is instantly available and the simplest method of feeding the baby.

7. Breast-feeding is more economical.

The merits of artificial feedings are likewise several:

1. Experience shows that intelligent mothers who rigorously follow the instructions of the doctor in the preparation of bottles and formula rarely meet difficulty in feeding their babies artificially.

2. The formula is always constant in composition and quantity; there is hence no question as to whether the

milk on any particular day is adequate for the baby's needs. On the contrary, the quantity of breast milk varies not only from day to day but from feeding to feeding, being most plentiful in the morning, least in the afternoon.

3. Despite the manipulations involved in preparation of the formula, artificial feeding is less tiring to the mother and she often regains her strength more rapidly. As they say, "it takes less out of her." Moreover, the early morning bottle, or a night bottle, may be given by the husband, or other third party, while the mother sleeps.

4. It is generally believed that the mother who feeds her baby artificially is in a better position to control her weight, regain her youthful figure and avoid sagging breasts. If viewed with some perspective, the validity of this statement is dubious. With exercise, carefully gauged diet and a properly fitting nursing brassière, the end results under the two methods of feeding should be the same.

5. If the mother is employed, artificial feeding offers unquestioned advantages.

It is barely possible that the above appraisal overstates the merits of artificial feeding, but despite this, it must be obvious that the advantages of breast-feeding, in so far as the baby is concerned, are considerable. In so far as the health of the mother is concerned, she will probably fare as well under one regime as under the other; as for her convenience, this will depend on individual circumstances. Returning now to our original questions, the following answers seem inescapable.

Should you nurse your baby? The answer is "Yes, if at all possible." Must you nurse your baby? The answer is "No, if circumstances make it quite impossible." The woman who is able to nurse her baby should consider herself fortunate. On the other hand, the woman who is unable to do so can rest assured that artificial feeding, if meticulously carried out, will usually yield results which are equally good.

Rooming-in. — By "rooming-in" is meant a program in which the infant is kept in a crib at the mother's bedside rather than in the nursery. It is an outgrowth in part of getting mothers up early, which permits the mother to be on her feet the second day and so take care of the baby herself. It stems in part also from the modern trend to make all phases of childbearing as "natural" as possible and to foster proper mother-child relationships at an early date. By the end of 24 hours the mother is generally out of bed; and thereafter, in this regime, she conducts under supervision by the nursery nurses most of the care of the infant. The mother thus becomes acquainted through actual experience with routine baby care.

Rooming-in, in varying degrees, is now being used in a number of hospitals. But in many institutions the architectural layout makes it impractical because the distance from the nursery to the patients' rooms is such that it is difficult for the nursery nurses (who look after the baby) to provide adequate supervision. Moreover, many doctors, perhaps the majority, disapprove of rooming-in in the belief that mothers need as much rest as possible at this time and should not be asked to shoulder the responsibilities of baby care during the first few days. Many mothers of experience hold a similar opinion, feeling that they get "rooming-in" soon enough when they go home.

HYGIENE OF THE PUERPERIUM

Diet. — After the first twenty-four hours, sometimes sooner, the majority of mothers are able to resume regular diet. With the birth of the baby, its demands upon the mother for nourishment do not end; they merely assume another form and continue to increase with the growth of the child. If the mother is to nurse adequately, therefore, the diet should be a generous and well-balanced one, amplified by milk or cocoa between meals and at bedtime. It is equally important that fluid intake should be substantial, not only because fluids are needed in milk formation, but also because they are excreted in unusual amounts at this time in the form of perspiration. The optimal fluid intake for a nursing mother is three to four quarts daily, one in the form of milk. Alcoholic drinks in small amounts (one drink) are harmless.

Bowels. — Constipation is the rule for two or three weeks after delivery, but as soon as normal activity is resumed, the condition disappears. Your physician will order suitable laxatives or enemas as necessary.

Bladder. — The majority of women have no difficulty with urination in the puerperium, but occasionally the neck of the bladder is unavoidably compressed as the baby is born and as a consequence the patient is unable to urinate. Sometimes very simple measures, which the nurse will suggest, suffice to relieve the difficulty — measures such as allowing water to run in the wash bowl, or placing a little steaming, hot water in the bedpan before use. If these, or similar procedures, are ineffectual, catheterization becomes necessary, that is, the urine is drained off by means of a small rubber tube inserted into the bladder. It may be necessary to repeat catheterization for several days; if so, the procedure becomes something of a nuisance, but it is painless and need cause no concern.

Abdominal Binder. — A snug binder applied to the abdomen after delivery often promotes the patient's comfort by relieving a certain sense of emptiness. Although physicians hold different views in regard to the desirability of such a binder, many favor it and few hold serious objections to its use, if requested by the patient.

Visitors. — In the seventeenth century, François Mauriceau, the great Parisian obstetrician of that epoch, wrote as follows:

> The Citizens Wives have a very ill Custom, which they would do well to refrain, that is, they cause their Children to be baptized the second or third Day after their labour; at which time all their Relations and Friends have a Collation in the Childbed Room, with whom she is obliged to discourse, and answer the Gossips, and all Comers a whole Afternoon together, with the usual Compliments of those Ceremonies, enough to distract her; and *tho' there is scarce any of the Company, which do not drink*

her Health, yet by the Noise they make in her Ears, she loses it.

I have taken the liberty of italicizing the last lines of Mauriceau's statement, since they epitomize what happens to countless young mothers today, as the result of continual salutations by well-intentioned friends. At no time is rest and quiet more needed than in the early days of the puerperium; and you yourself will realize, when the time comes, how draining it is to have to perk up and receive friend after friend (and relative after relative), all bubbling over with congratulations. During the first three days, visitors should be restricted to husband, parents, and possibly an intimate friend or two. While more latitude is permissible subsequently, even then it is judicious to curtail the number of visitors to two or three a day. As Mrs. Helen Washburn remarks in her delightful book, *So You're Going to Have a Baby*, "You don't have to bother to explain to them about this. Nurses are expert at throwing people out. They love it."

Then too, you must remember that nursing schedule and face the fact that your night's rest is no longer what it used to be. Accordingly a daily nap is imperative. Indeed, throughout the entire puerperium, the hours between two and four in the afternoon should be reserved for a complete rest.

The "Baby Blues." — There are sound scientific grounds for believing that the nervous system after delivery is more sensitive than at other times. Even if this were not so, it would be surprising if this long-anticipated event of childbirth, so epoch-making to the young woman, so far-reaching in its ramifications, did not occasionally evoke profound emotional responses. Most common among such reactions, perhaps, is what is colloquially called the "Baby Blues." About the time that everything is going perfectly in the puerperium, with mother and baby both flourishing and everybody happy, the mother, for no accountable reason, bursts into a good, long cry. Nothing can stop her; persuasion is futile; she simply continues to sob and weep for a good half hour. When the episodes is over, she can offer no explanation. "It just came over me," she says. Such reactions rarely recur and following them the mother usually feels much better. In view of all that has taken place during the past nine months, it requires no psychiatrist to interpret episodes of this kind, but simply an understanding heart.

Afterpains. — Occasionally menstrual-like cramps are experienced during the first three days of the puerperium by women who have had previous children; after first babies, they are met less frequently. These so-called "afterpains" are due, as a rule, to the presence of small clots in the uterus and result from the contractions made by the uterus in its effort to expel these. They are likely to be particularly pronounced when the baby nurses, because of the connection which exists between the breasts and uterus (page 178). They are of no serious moment, but if at all severe, the doctor should be advised so that medication may be prescribed.

Cracked Nipples. — A large number of mothers, perhaps one half, complain of sore nipples during the early days of nursing. This condition is usually ascribable either to small cracks in the nipple or to raw areas. In the event nursing becomes painful, the fact should be reported to the doctor at once for it is important that early treatment be started. Various healing ointments may be employed to allay the irritation and ordinarily the disturbance responds readily. Since the baby's tugging at the nipple tends to prolong the irritation, the doctor may advise temporary suspension of nursing and the use, meanwhile, of a nipple shield or a breast pump. A nipple shield is a round, glass cup which fits tightly around the outer edge of the nipple; attached to it is a rubber nipple which the child nurses. In this way the child's mouth is prevented from coming in direct contact with the nipple. A similar device is applied to the nipple when pumping is employed, artificial suction being derived either from a rubber bulb or from an electric-suction apparatus. Under most circumstances the milk secured by pumping may be given to the baby in a bottle. After such measures as this have given the nipple a rest for twenty-four to forty-eight hours, direct nursing can usually be resumed without further discomfort.

Getting Up and Going Home. — The first day up, the mother simply sits in a chair for half an hour, morning and afternoon; walking is ordinarily begun the second day up and increased until the patient is able to be on her feet for five or ten minutes without fatigue. She is then, as a rule, allowed to go home.

As the result of dire shortages in hospital beds the country over, it has become customary to get mothers up earlier and send them home sooner than was formerly done; and physicians everywhere (and mothers too) have been pleasantly surprised at the results of this accelerated program — particularly with the greater rapidity with which strength is regained. Depending on circumstances, patients nowadays stay in bed only from one to three days after delivery. The time of going home varies between the fourth and tenth day, as a rule; the average is near the fifth or sixth.

In this connection, there is no greater boon to the young mother just home from the hospital than a nurse. Practical nurses are altogether satisfactory for this purpose and are much cheaper than trained nurses. Even if such a nurse can be had for only a few days, she will be of immeasurable value to the mother during this period of readjustment. Be sure to ask your doctor about the availability of such nurses.

It is well to recall, during these early days at home, that the pelvic organs do not return to normal until six or more weeks after delivery and that strength returns, only gradually, over a corresponding interval. Do not expect to become a bundle of energy within a few short weeks. During the first two weeks at home it is best to remain on one floor and during the third to limit stairclimbing to a minimum. Mothers rarely regain their full vigor and "feel their old self" again until the baby is almost two months old.

Exercises. — In order that the abdominal muscles, as well as other structures concerned in pregnancy and labor, may be restored to normal as completely and rapidly as possible, many doctors recommend that the patient perform certain exercises in the puerperium. Some physicians start very simple muscular movements a day or two after delivery, while others prefer to wait until a week or ten days have passed. Since the optimal time to begin such activity depends on the circumstances of delivery, and other considerations, the patient should never undertake exercising without specific instructions from her doctor. The following three exercises are particularly helpful in correcting flabbiness of the abdominal wall and in removing excess fat from the upper thighs, hips and abdomen.

1. Lie flat on your back and raise the right foot a few inches off the bed, keeping the leg stiff; lower it slowly. Do the same with the left leg. Using each leg alternately, repeat eight times, or a fewer number if fatigued. Each day or two endeavor to raise the leg higher and higher until it is possible, without tiring, to raise each eight times to a perpendicular position. When this can be accomplished with ease, probably several weeks after delivery, raise both legs several inches off the bed (or floor), keeping the legs stiff and together. This is much more difficult. Gradually, nevertheless, increase the height to which the legs are elevated until it is possible to raise both legs simultaneously, not only to the perpendicular position, but further, so that your toes are directly over your head. Repeat eight times (Figure 10).

2. Lie flat on your back with the arms folded across the chest. Raise your head off the pillow a few inches. Repeat eight times. Gradually increase the height to

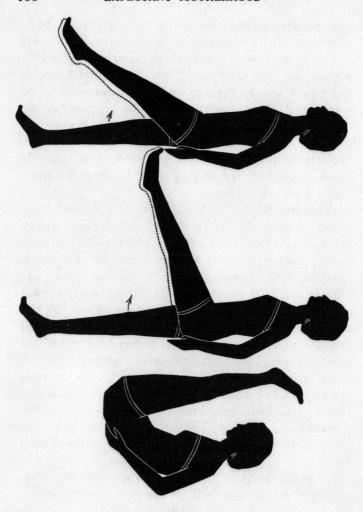

Figure 10. Leg-Raising Exercise.

which the head is raised until you are able (a number of weeks after delivery) to rise to a sitting position, with the arms folded across the chest (Figure 11).

3. Lie flat on your back and raise the hips off the bed a few inches. With the hips thus elevated, contract the muscles around the rectum in the same manner in which

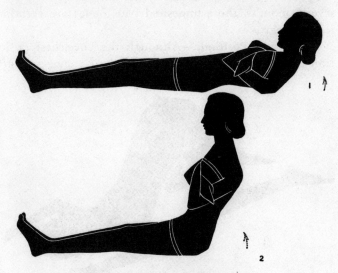

Figure 11. Sitting-Up Exercise.

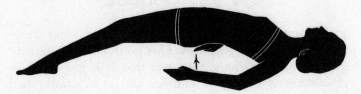

Figure 12. Hip-Raising Exercise.

a bowel movement is held back. Now return to the lying posture. As time goes on, increase the height to which the hips are raised and the force with which the muscles around the rectum are contracted (Figure 12).

With persistence, exercise of this sort will work wonders. Nothing can be accomplished in a few days, or even in a few weeks, but if the exercises are kept up for several months, those undesired pads of fat are certain to disappear.

Knee-Chest Position. — Although the knee-chest position is not an exercise, your physician may suggest that

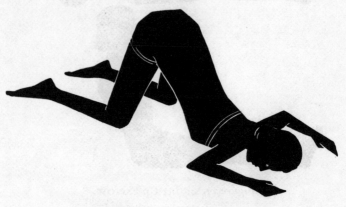

Figure 13. Knee-Chest Position.

you assume this posture for five minutes night and morning after you go home. This position is illustrated in Figure 13. It should be noted that it is not a knee-*elbow,* but a knee-*chest* position; in other words, the head must be turned one way or the other, while the elbows are allowed to fall to the side. The knees should be twelve to eighteen inches apart, permitting air to enter the vagina. The entrance of air into the vagina, indeed, is the aim of the procedure since this causes the uterus to fall forward in such a position that the circulation in the pelvic organs is improved.

Resumption of Tub Baths. — Tub baths are permissible for the mother, as a rule, when the baby is three weeks old. If desired, showers may be taken as soon as the mother can stand firmly on her feet.

Intercourse. — It is judicious to defer intercourse until two full months after delivery.

Final Examination. — Some doctors make it a practice to carry out a careful pelvic examination on patients just before they leave the hospital. Almost all request that the patient return to the office for a final check-up when the baby is between six weeks and two months old. At this time, as a rule, the mother can be assured that complete restitution of her pelvic organs has occurred and that her normal regime may be resumed. Occasionally, minor deviations from the normal are encountered and, if so, future trouble can be forestalled by suitable treatment at this time.

Return of Menstruation. — In women who do not nurse their infants, menstruation usually returns within four to eight weeks after delivery, but it may not return until three or four months. Since lactation ordinarily tends to inhibit menstruation, the majority of women who nurse their babies do not menstruate for some five or six months; and not infrequently, menstruation is absent as long as lactation continues. There is great individual variation, however, and occasionally a woman will menstruate despite the fact that she is nursing her baby.

The first menstrual period after childbirth is almost always abnormal in one respect or another. It is often profuse, with clots, and may stop and later start again. This is the rule and should be of no concern. The second period is usually normal.

Activities. — Your doctor will not object to your going out and driving your car if you wish, after you have been home from the hospital three weeks.

You may shampoo your hair when desired (a question often asked).

Chapter XI

THE NEWBORN BABY

ALTHOUGH the mother has no direct responsibility for the care of her baby during the first week or so of the puerperium, she will naturally want to acquaint herself with all that concerns this new and precious possession. As soon as the baby is born, or within a few seconds, he puckers his lips into a cry and generally wails lustily for a number of minutes. The abundance of air thus breathed in serves the important purpose of enriching the infant's blood with oxygen and consequently his color becomes a bright pink. The doctor now ties and cuts the umbilical cord, and forthwith the baby is launched into life as a separate individual.

As late as half a century ago, about one third of all patients in blind asylums owed their blindness to infections which they had contracted at birth; in the vast majority of cases the cause was gonorrhea, but it is known that other types of infection may also be responsible. In 1884, a great German obstetrician, Karl Credé, discovered that a drop or two of a weak silver-nitrate solution dropped into each eye immediately after birth assured healthy eyes. This was one of the most beneficent contributions ever made to medicine, for its employment has almost eliminated this cruel scourge. It is now a law in most states that the doctor must instill some kind of silver solution into the eyes of every baby shortly after birth. Now, however, a solution of penicillin, or penicillin ointment, is being used in some hospitals instead of a silver preparation. The antiseptic solution itself may occasionally cause mild irritation for a day or two; accordingly, if your baby develops some redness of its eyelids, along with a small amount of secretion, do not think that this portends a cold or an infection, but understand that it is merely a slight chemical irritation which is invariably harmless and of brief duration.

After the eyes have been treated and a suitable dressing put on the cord, the nurse places the baby in a warm corner of the delivery room and gives it its first bath. In some hospitals this takes the form of an oil bath with warm mineral oil; in others, warm water and a bland soap are used. In many hospitals no bath whatsoever is given in the belief that the vernix caseosa (page 37) is the best protective dressing that the baby's skin can have. At this time (before either mother or baby leaves the delivery room), some unmistakable identifying label is affixed to the baby; this may consist of a string of lettered beads around the ankle, spelling out the mother's name, or a piece of adhesive tape applied to the baby's back with the mother's name printed on it, or both. In any event, the mother may rest assured that the most meticulous labeling of each baby, before either mother or baby leaves the delivery room, is now a routine part of its hospital care, and that the old bugaboo of many a mother, "mixed babies," can be dismissed into the limbo of bad dreams. Following the bath, the baby is dressed in diapers, shirt and gown, and placed in a warm crib.

What is it like, this new, tiny creature?

Weight. — There are invariably two questions which are asked at once by every mother, husband and relative: Is it a boy or a girl? How much does it weigh? The former query, of course, can be answered immediately. The latter, depending on the custom of the hospital, may require an hour or two, since some institutions (and some doctors) prefer to postpone weighing the baby until it has had time to become adjusted to its new environment. If the baby is very small (premature), it may not be weighed for a day or two. Many hospitals use the metric system in weighing babies and report their weight in grams. While any doctor or nurse will be glad to convert this figure into pounds for you, you can do it yourself if you multiply the weight in grams by 22 and then mark off four decimal places from the right; in other words, multiply by .0022. For example, if the weight of the baby is 3000 grams, .0022 times 3000 equals 6.6000 pounds, that is, six and six tenths pounds, or six pounds and two thirds. In following the weight gain of the baby from day to day — if reported in grams — it will be helpful to recall that thirty grams is about one ounce. (Actually, 28.35 grams equal one ounce.)

Infants born at full term average about seven and one quarter pounds in weight, boys weighing usually about three ounces more than girls. Healthy newborn infants may range from five pounds to eleven pounds. A weight of less than five pounds ordinarily signifies that the baby has been born ahead of time and is referred to as a "premature" infant.

During the few days before the milk comes in, the baby undergoes a weight loss which averages about 7 per cent of its birth weight; in the case of a seven-pound baby this would mean approximately one half pound. Although this loss is entirely normal and is readily regained, some doctors give the baby sugar water or other solutions the first three days in order to offset it; not a few competent specialists, on the other hand, question the desirability of this procedure. Most babies make up this loss rapidly and are back at their birth weight by the tenth or twelfth day. With the exception of premature infants, babies are generally weighed daily when in the hospital. In the event there is any question about the amount of milk the baby is receiving, it may also be weighed before and after nursing.

Length. — The average newborn baby is about twenty inches long, boys tending to be somewhat longer than girls.

Bodily Contour. — A newborn infant is by no means simply the miniature of an adult, but is a creature unto itself and differs from the adult in many, many ways. Its head is proportionately large, representing about one quarter of the body length; likewise, its abdomen is very prominent. On the other hand, the chest is narrow and the limbs short. The legs (which in a few years will be as straight as an arrow) are so markedly bowed that the soles of the feet may nearly face each other. The neck is short because of the abundance of fat in this region. To the dismay of many parents, the baby's head is often distinctly lopsided during the first fortnight and may even have a large, dome-shaped lump on one side or the other. This asymmetry is due to the compression and molding which the head undergoes in passing through the birth canal; it is temporary and will disappear in a week or so. Because of the large size of the head, and the weak neck muscles, the baby cannot hold its head up alone and hence the head must always be supported until the infant is about three months old. The bones which make up the skull of the newborn are not joined together, but have soft membranous spaces between them. One of these spaces is quite large and may be felt as a soft, diamond-shaped depression just above the forehead. The bones surrounding this "fontanelle," as physicians call it, gradually close in, but the space is not completely obliterated until the infant is about eighteen months old.

Skin. — The color of the skin varies from pink to deep red. Tiny, scarcely visible white spots are often seen on the face, particularly about the nose, but these are of no significance and disappear in a short time. The sweat glands are inactive at birth and for about a month afterward, and consequently the baby does not perspire at this period — a wise provision on the part of Nature to conserve body heat and body fluids. About the third or fourth day, the skin may assume a yellowish tinge; this jaundice of the newborn is very common and is regarded by those who have studied the phenomenon as a perfectly normal reaction of the baby's bodily economy to its new environment. It is of no consequence and disappears between the seventh and tenth days. It is scarcely necessary to add that the skin of the newborn is very sensitive and throughout the early months diaper rashes, as well as skin irritations from various causes, are common. Although these disturbances are generally minor in character, they should be reported to your physician, for early treatment usually means early cure.

Hair. — The scalp at birth is covered by a variable amount of fine, silky hair, usually black. About the beginning of the second week this begins to fall out and often the head is left almost bald. Gradually new hair appears and, as a rule, this is firmer in texture and of lighter color. In other words, the appearance of the baby's hair at birth gives little clue as to what its character will be later on.

Nails. — The finger- and toenails are perfectly developed. The former often extend slightly beyond the ends of the fingers, and to prevent the baby's scratching himself, it is often necessary for the nurse to clip the nails early in life. As she will explain to you, it is easiest to do this when the baby is asleep.

Eyes and Ears. — The eyes of the newborn are peculiar in several respects. The eyebrows and eyelashes are barely discernible, being extremely short and fine. Since the tear-producing apparatus is not yet active, there are no tears at this time, no matter how lustily the baby may cry, and these do not develop for several weeks; they are well established by the second month, however, and then, as if to make up for lost time — but you will find out for yourself in the due course of years. Another characteristic feature of every newborn baby's eyes is their utter lack of co-ordination. Indeed, they roll around to all corners of the compass until every new mother is certain that her child is going to be cross-eyed. Recalling that the eye muscles have had no use in the uterus, it is understandable that they are weak at birth; with time and use they will strengthen. Light perception is present at birth, but little information can be obtained concerning actual sight. Unquestionably, it becomes developed within a few days or weeks. Hearing is probably present very shortly after birth, since the baby will respond to noises within the first week.

Breasts. — Boy babies, as well as girls, often exhibit a marked swelling and hardness of the breasts during the first week; and occasionally, a small amount of secretion can be expressed from the nipple. This is called "witch's milk" and in medieval times this strange fluid was thought to have miraculous healing powers. The phenomenon is attributable to the fact that the same substance which causes the mother's breasts to enlarge in pregnancy passes through the placenta and exerts a similar effect on the breasts of the infant in the uterus. The swelling usually subsides by the end of the first week.

Pseudo-Menstruation. — "Pseudo" or false menstruation is seen in about one girl baby in twenty; it generally amounts to little more than a slight spotting of the diaper with blood for a few days. Here, again, is a condition attributable to the passage of a certain substance through the placenta, that same substance which built up the lining membrane of the mother's uterus in preparation for pregnancy (pages 19-22). All these months this substance has acted on the infant's uterus so that its lining also becomes very thick. As soon as the baby is born, this substance, which was received from the mother, of course, is withdrawn and the thickened lining of the baby's uterus collapses; as a result, a slight amount of bleeding occasionally ensues.

Umbilical Cord. — Since the bulk of the umbilical cord is composed of a watery, jellylike substance, which surrounds the blood vessels within, the cord dries up readily when exposed to air. After the doctor cuts and ties it following delivery, a small section of an inch or so is left attached to the abdomen of the baby. This stump begins to shrivel the first day or two after birth and by the end of the first week, it is reduced to a small fraction of its former thickness, being little more than a dry, black string. The time at which this remnant of the cord falls off varies greatly; it may separate as early as the seventh day or as late as the sixteenth or eighteenth day; the average time is around the tenth or twelfth day. This process rarely gives rise to difficulty but in the event the cord should still be attached when the mother leaves the hospital, the physician or nurses will give instructions about its care.

Bowels. — During the first two or three days, the stools consist of a greenish-black, tarry material, called "meconium." This represents various products which have accumulated in the intestine before birth. After the third day, the stools assume a lighter shade and are shortly golden-yellow in color and pasty in consistency. During the first month of life, babies have from one to four stools a day.

Circumcision. — Oddly enough, the two oldest surgical operations known are both performed on the newborn infant. One of these is the cutting of the umbilical cord; the other is circumcision, or the cutting off of the foreskin of male babies. Circumcision has been carried out as a religious rite or tribal custom since prehistoric times and is still practiced, of course, by most Semitic peoples. From a medical viewpoint, there are two schools of thought in regard to this procedure. Some doctors feel that it is judicious to circumcise every boy baby for purposes of cleanliness; certainly, if the infant is circumcised, washing of the genitals is much easier, for otherwise the foreskin has to be retracted at each bath. On the other hand, many physicians consider it preferable to circumcise only those infants in which the foreskin cannot be drawn back readily. Your doctor will give you advice on this question and, in case you and your husband request it, will perform the operation the day before you go home or perhaps earlier. The procedure is a minor one and, when done by a doctor, rarely gives rise to the slightest disturbance.

Sleep. — During the first two weeks, the baby sleeps most of the time, that is, twenty to twenty-two hours a day. At this period, indeed, he seems to have but two interests, sleeping and eating. The suckling reflex is marvelously developed and, even a few minutes after birth, he will immediately suckle any objects put to his lips.

Premature Infants. — When a baby is born a month or more ahead of the expected date of confinement, he is handicapped in various ways. In the first place, the development of his various organs is not quite complete and accordingly, he is less well equipped to cope with conditions outside of the uterus; for instance, his lungs, nervous system and digestive organs are feebler and they may have difficulty in carrying out their functions. He faces another disadvantage in the fact that he has little body fat. It will be recalled that the baby acquires most of the fat on its body during the last month in the uterus. This fat is most important in keeping the body warm and in its absence, the problem of maintaining body heat in a premature infant is sometimes most difficult. Finally, the premature baby is much more subject to infection than the full-term child.

Despite these handicaps, meticulous care is making it possible to rear an increasing number of these small babies, particularly if they weigh more than four pounds. The prospect for infants who weigh less than this amount is always dubious and when their weight is two pounds or under, the outlook is almost hopeless. The smallest premature baby which has been raised weighed in the neighborhood of a pound and a half, but such good fortune is extremely rare.

Twins. — Twins occur once in eighty births, approximately; triplets once in 6400 births; and quadruplets once in half a million. Over thirty cases of quintuplets have been recorded, but with rare exceptions, none of these infants has survived more than a few weeks. The most notable exception, of course, is the Dionne quintuplets, and the fact that all five of these girls successfully survived infancy and childhood is one of the miracles of modern times. As is well known, heredity plays an important causative role in twin pregnancy; and if there are already twins in the family of the expectant mother, or in that of the husband, the likelihood of twins is decidedly greater.

Twins may be of two kinds, like and unlike, or to phrase it differently, identical and nonidentical. Identical twins *are* identical because they come from a single egg; fertilization takes place in the usual way, by a single spermatozoon, but then, very early in the egg's development, it divides into two identical parts instead of continuing as a single individual. Such twins are always of the same sex and, as we have already implied, show close physical and mental resemblances. Unlike, or nonidentical, twins come from the fertilization of two eggs by two spermatozoa. Such twins, according to chance, may be of the same sex or of opposite sexes; and the likelihood of their resembling each other is no greater than that of any brother and sister. These unlike twins are much the more common of the two types, making up about 70 per cent of all twins.

In the majority of instances (but not all), it is possible for the physician to make a diagnosis of twins by abdominal examination during the last few months; in doubtful cases an X-ray picture may be necessary to settle the question. The latter weeks of a twin pregnancy usually impose more discomfort on the mother than carrying a single child; heaviness of the lower abdomen, back pains and swelling of the feet and ankles may be particularly troublesome. For this, and other reasons, it is highly important that a woman with a twin pregnancy follow her doctor's instructions with rigid care.

Twins are likely to be born about two weeks before the calculated date of confinement — a fact which should be taken into consideration in making plans. Even though the pregnancy goes to full term, twin babies are usually smaller than single infants by nearly a pound; however, the outlook for such babies, provided that the pregnancy continues into the last month, is almost as good as that for single infants.

Birth Certificate. — Three or four weeks after delivery, you will receive at your residence address the birth certificate of the baby. This is issued by the local health department on data which your doctor or the hospital has supplied. If it has not arrived at the end of two months, so inform your doctor who will inquire into the reason for the delay. This document may someday prove of the utmost value to your child and it should be preserved most carefully.

Care of the Baby at Home. — Going home with the new baby is always something of a gala occasion and it should be, for it marks the beginning of a new phase in the life of both mother and child. The baby, now adjusted to conditions outside the mother's body, is ready to embark on the routine life of babyhood; while the mother, in large measure restored to her previous state, is prepared to take over its care.

During the last day or two in the hospital, the mother should take opportunity to watch the nurse bathe the baby, prepare its water bottle, and if a formula is needed, she should learn exactly how it is prepared. She will doubtless receive other valuable advice from the nurses about the general care of the baby at home. Here, however, as in pregnancy, the mother's chief guidebook must be the physician. It may be that the doctor who attended you at delivery will also care for your baby at home; or, very possibly, he may turn over its supervision to a specialist, that is, to a pediatrician. But whoever your baby doctor may be, it is highly desirable that he take the baby under his surveillance during your stay in the hospital. After examining it carefully, he will explain in detail everything you will need to know: food, clothes, habits and care; and once this alliance is established, he will never be farther away from your child than the nearest telephone. Beyond question, such an arrangement is the surest guarantee of a healthy baby and a worry-free mother.

INDEX